HOW TO BE CARNIVORE

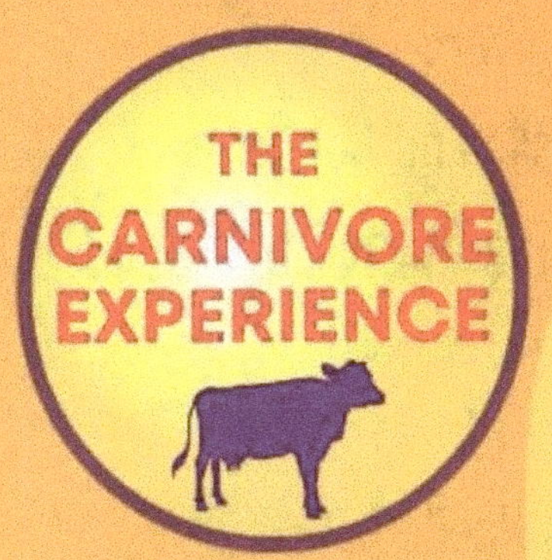

Stephen Thomas BSc. (Hons.)

Table Of Contents

The Carnivore Experience

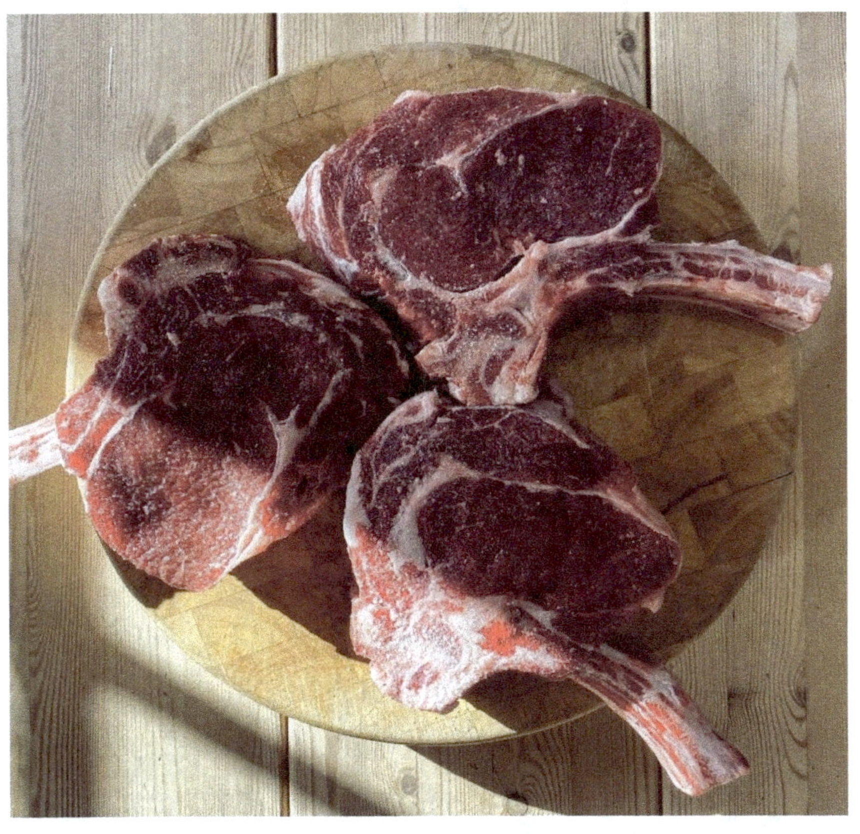

Chapter 1: Understanding the Carnivore Diet

What is the Carnivore Diet?

The Carnivore Way Of Eating is a dietary approach that involves consuming only animal products such as meat, fish, eggs, and dairy while avoiding all plant-based foods. This diet is gaining popularity among people looking to improve their health and body composition due to its potential benefits for weight loss, improved energy levels, and overall well-being.

The basic principle behind the Carnivore Diet is that humans are primarily carnivorous animals and that our bodies are better adapted to digesting and utilizing animal products as opposed to plant-based foods. By eliminating all plant foods from your diet, you are removing potential sources of inflammation, allergens, and anti-nutrients that can negatively impact your health.

Many people who have adopted the Carnivore Diet have reported significant improvements in their health, including weight loss, increased energy levels, better digestion, and reduced inflammation. You may have seen numerous success stories interviews on various social media platforms, including my own channel. By focusing on nutrient-dense animal foods, you can provide your body with essential nutrients such as protein, fats, vitamins, and minerals that are crucial for optimal health and well-being.

If you are considering starting the Carnivore Diet, it is important to do your research, which is possibly why you are reading this book? It is also important to listen to your body and make adjustments as needed to ensure that you are meeting your nutritional needs while following the Carnivore Diet.

In the next chapters of "How To Be Carnivore: Your Roadmap to Better Health," we will dive deeper into the principles of the Carnivore Diet, provide practical tips for getting started, and share delicious recipes to help you on your journey to better health and body composition. For further exploration and enhanced learning, readers are encouraged to utilize the website www.theukcarnivore.com and The Carnivore Experience app as they are valuable supplementary resources that complement and illustrate the content discussed in the book.

Study: Carnivore For Health

Throughout the book I will include various studies. Feel free to skip these if the science is not why you bought this book.

Contrary to common expectations, adults consuming a carnivore diet experienced few adverse effects and instead reported health benefits and high satisfaction.

https://www.ncbi.nlm.nih.gov/pmc/articles/PMC8684475/

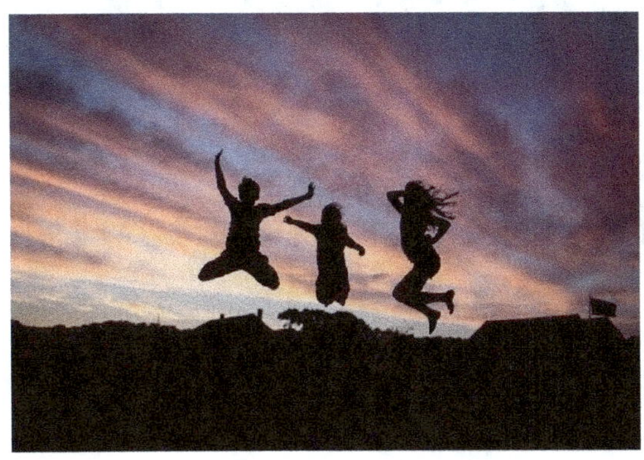

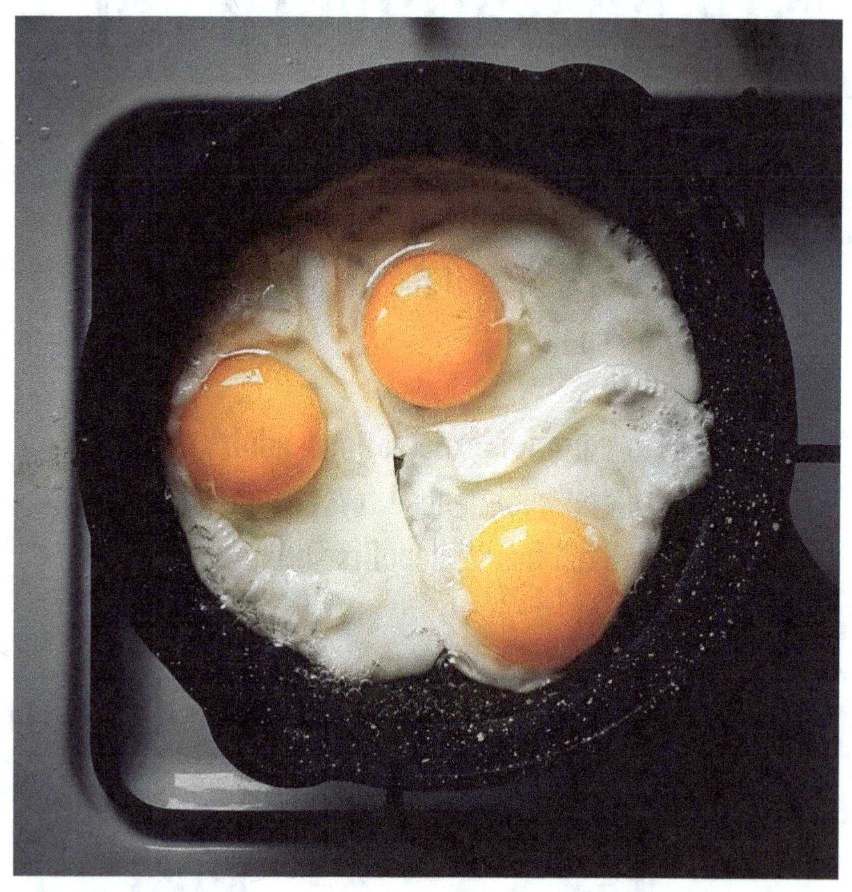

Benefits of the Carnivore Diet

In this subchapter, we will dive into the numerous benefits of the carnivore diet for those looking to improve their health and body composition. The carnivore diet, which consists of primarily animal-based foods such as meat, fish, poultry and eggs, has gained popularity in recent years for its potential to optimize health and help individuals achieve their desired body composition goals.

One of the key benefits of the carnivore diet is its ability to promote body fat loss. By eliminating carbohydrates and focusing on protein and healthy fats, the carnivore diet can help regulate hunger hormones and promote a state of satiety, making it easier to adhere to healthy eating and lose excess body fat. By eating foods that keep blood glucose stable and does not tend to raise insulin in 'spikes,' the carnivore diet has been beneficial for those looking to lose body fat, control their diabetes or both.

In summary, the carnivore diet has been shown to improve metabolic health markers such as blood sugar levels, insulin sensitivity, and other markers of good health. By eliminating processed foods, grains, pasta, rice, breads and sugars, the carnivore diet can help reduce inflammation in the body and improve overall metabolic function.

Many individuals also report increased energy levels and mental clarity when following the carnivore diet. By providing the body with a steady source of high-quality nutrients and eliminating potential food sensitivities, the carnivore diet can help improve cognitive function and overall well-being.

Furthermore, the carnivore diet is known for its simplicity and ease of adherence. With a focus on animal-based foods, the carnivore diet eliminates the need for complicated meal planning and can be easily tailored to individual preferences and dietary restrictions.

Overall, the carnivore diet offers a range of benefits for those looking to improve their health and body composition. By focusing on nutrient-dense animal foods and eliminating processed carbohydrates, the carnivore diet can help individuals achieve their health and fitness goals in a sustainable and effective manner.

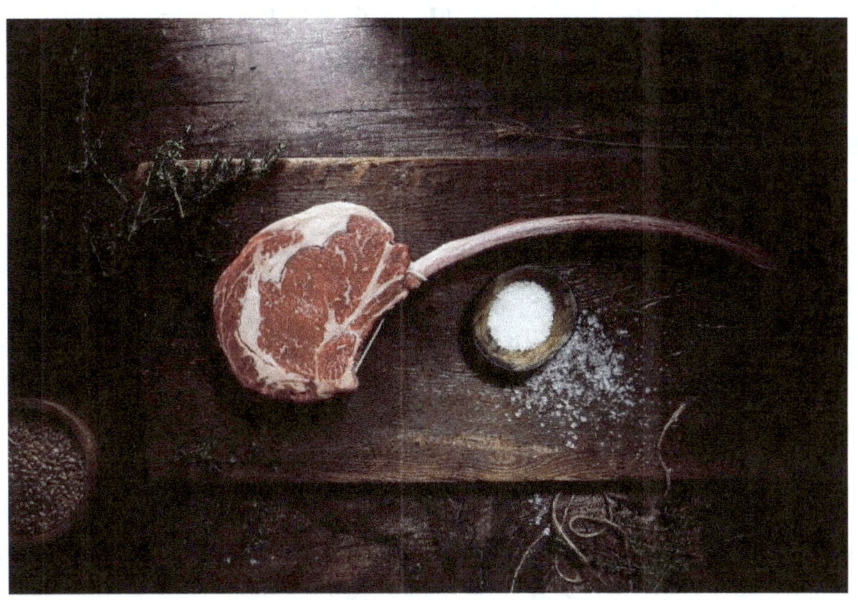

Study: Safe Carnivore

The safety of a Carnivore Diet raises no concerns.

Throughout the entirety of human evolution, which commenced around 4 million years ago with the Australopithecus walking upright and hunting animals, our ancestors have been consuming animals. This has led some to argue that hunting animals played a pivotal role in facilitating the growth of our brains in size and complexity over the subsequent years.

https://www.pnas.org/doi/10.1073/pnas.1814087116

Exceptionally high $\delta15N$ values in collagen single amino acids confirm Neandertals as high-trophic level carnivores Klervia Jaouen klervia_jaouen@eva.mpg.de, Michael P. Richards https://orcid.org/0000-0001-5274-8887, Adeline Le Cabec https://orcid.org/0000-0001-6948-4726, +4, and Sahra Talamo

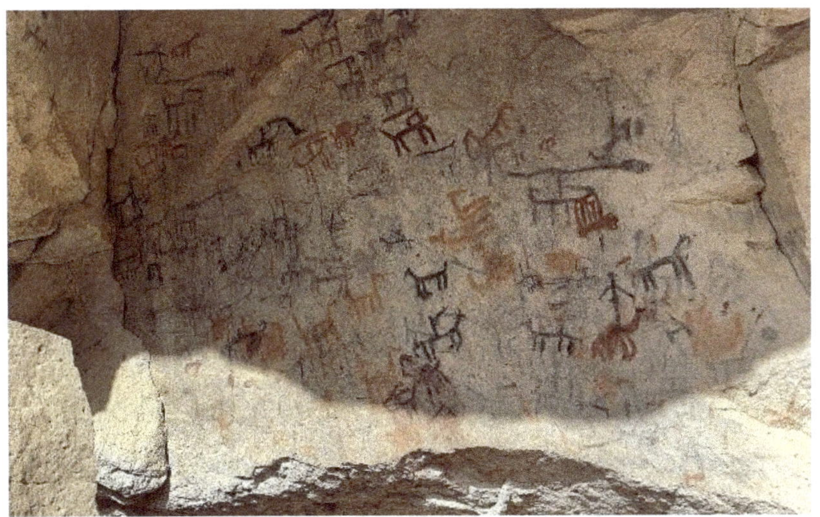

No cave painting depicting a human eating a salad has been discovered. The assertion that humans cannot be carnivores because they do not possess pointed teeth lacks common sense. Human beings do have pointed teeth called canines, and moreover, historical evidence indicates that humans did not use their teeth to attack animals; instead, they utilized their intellect and tools for hunting.

https://www.straitstimes.com/lifestyle/food/debunking-a-few-myths-about-meat-eating-and-vegetarianism

Potential Risks and Concerns

When starting the Carnivore Diet, it is important to be aware of the potential risks and concerns that may arise. While many people have experienced significant improvements in their health and body composition on this diet, there are some possible risks that should be considered.

Some people may experience difficulty adapting to the high-fat nature of the Carnivore Diet, especially if they are used to a low-fat diet. It is important to gradually increase your fat intake and listen to your body's hunger and fullness cues to ensure you are getting enough nutrition and energy from your meals.

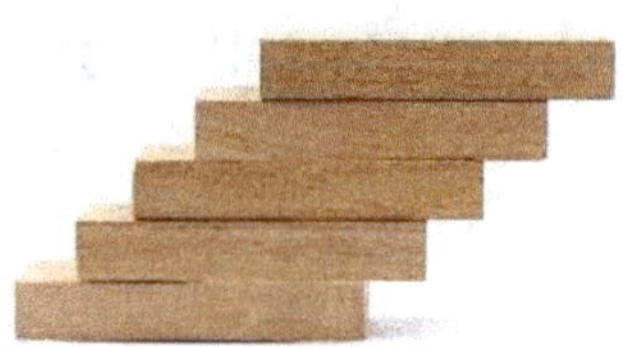

The Carnivore Experience

Overall, while the Carnivore Diet can offer many health benefits, it is important to be aware of the potential risks and concerns that may arise. By being mindful of eating enough, potential electrolyte imbalances due to reducing the body's excess water retention formed during a high carbohydrate diet, and adjusting to a higher fat diet, you can navigate these challenges and set yourself up for success on your journey to better health and body composition.

There is a handy troubleshooting page on my website
https://www.theukcarnivore.com/troubleshooting

Chapter 2: Getting Started with the Carnivore Diet

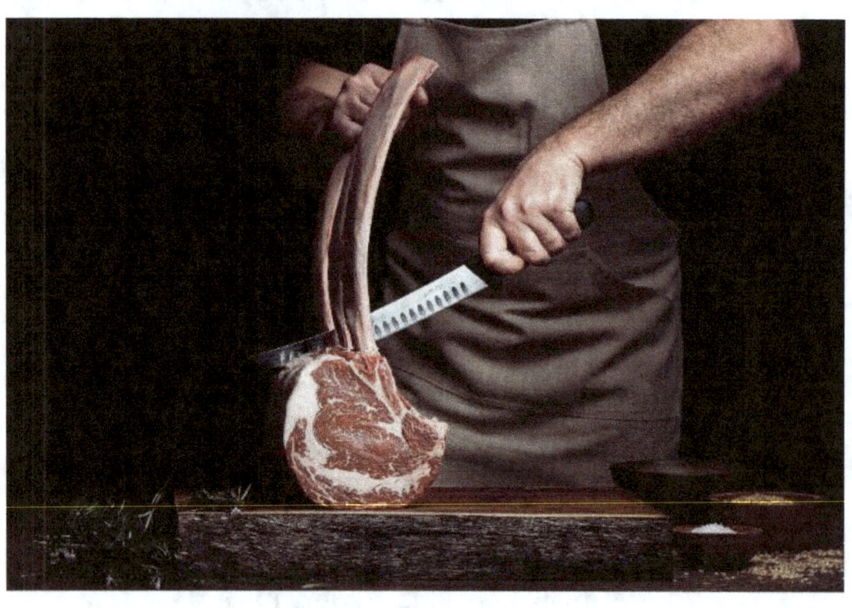

Preparing Your Mindset

Before embarking on the carnivore diet, it is crucial to prepare your mindset for the journey ahead. Changing your eating habits and lifestyle can be challenging, but with the right mindset, you can set yourself up for success. **Some people even claim you have to be 'ready,' before you start.** Here are some tips to help you prepare mentally for starting the carnivore diet:

1. Set clear goals: Before starting the carnivore diet, take some time to define your goals. Whether you want to improve your health, lose weight, or simply feel better, having clear goals will help you stay motivated and focused throughout your journey.

2. Educate yourself: Take the time to research the carnivore diet and understand the science behind it. Knowing the benefits of the diet and how it can improve your health and body composition will help you stay committed when faced with challenges. My website, app and YouTube channel have dedicated playlists such as 'ask the experts,' and 'science-based health and wellbeing.'

3. Stay positive: Changing your eating habits can be tough, but maintaining a positive attitude is key to success. Instead of focusing on what you can't eat, shift your mindset to all the delicious and nutritious foods you can enjoy on the carnivore diet.

4. Embrace the process: Remember that transitioning to the carnivore diet is a journey, not a destination. Be patient with yourself and allow yourself time to adjust to the new way of eating. Celebrate small victories along the way and don't get discouraged by setbacks.

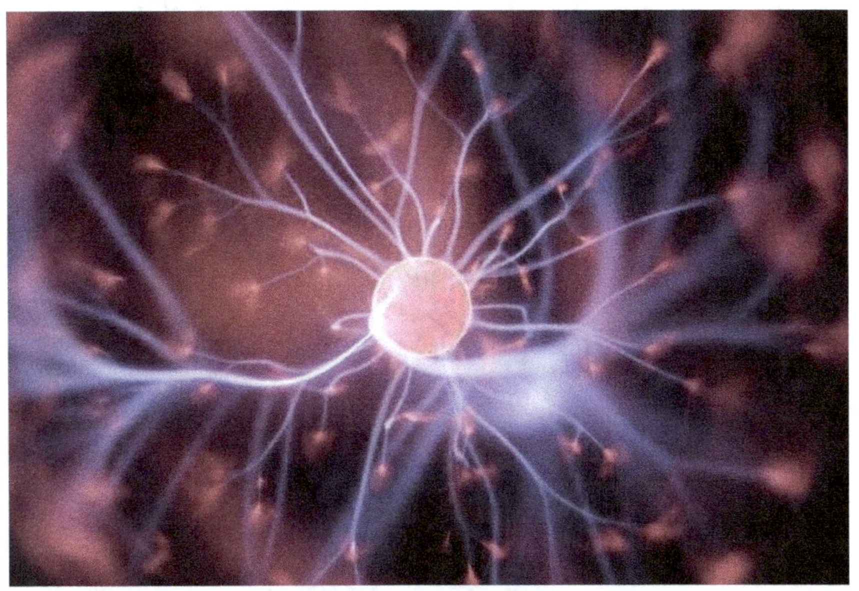

5. Seek support: Surround yourself with like-minded individuals who can support you on your carnivore diet journey. Join online communities, find a accountability partner, or seek guidance from a health coach or nutritionist specializing in the carnivore diet. I have a private Facebook group you could join as an example.

By preparing your mindset before starting the carnivore diet, you will set yourself up for success and be better equipped to overcome any challenges that may come your way. Remember, your mindset is just as important as your diet when it comes to improving your health and body composition.

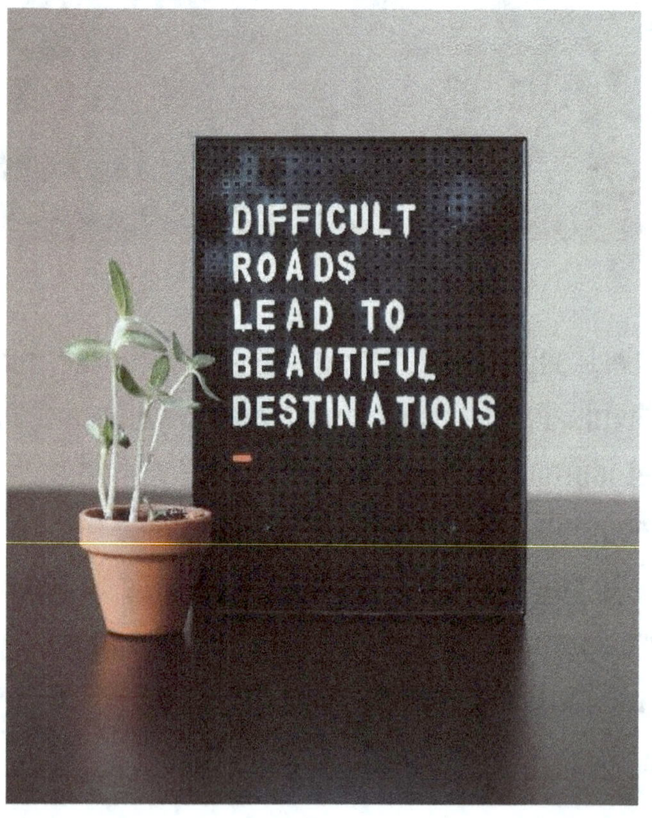

Study: No Carbs Needed

Carbohydrate is the only macronutrient with no established minimum requirement.

Although carbohydrates are the only food constituents that directly increase blood glucose (the main determinant of insulin secretion), population studies indicate that the type of carbohydrate plays a more significant role than the total amount of carbohydrate in the risk of chronic disease https://www.ncbi.nlm.nih.gov/pmc/articles/PMC5996878/ is text to edit.

Clearing Out Your Kitchen

One of the first steps to successfully starting the Carnivore Diet is to clear out your kitchen of any non-compliant foods. This may seem daunting at first, but it is crucial for setting yourself up for success on this journey to better health and body composition.

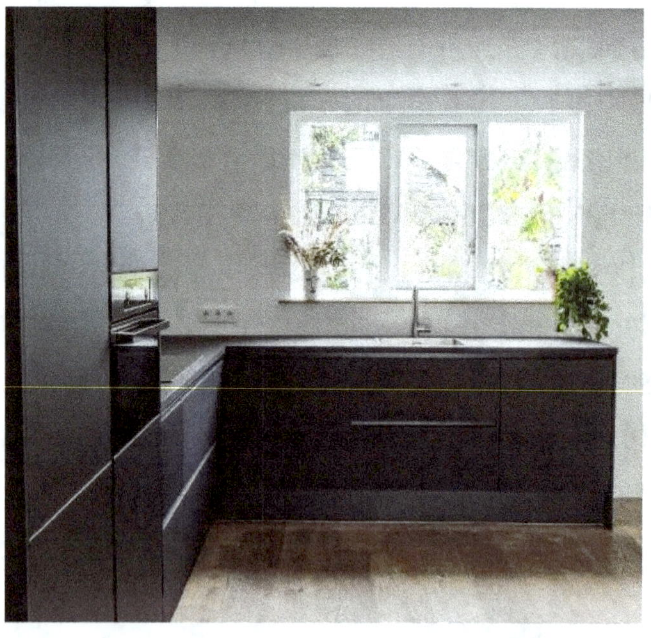

Start by removing all processed foods, grains, sugars, dairy products, and plant-based products from your pantry, refrigerator, and freezer. These foods are not part of the Carnivore Diet and can hinder your progress if they are readily available to you.

Next, take a closer look at ingredient labels on any packaged foods you may have. Many products contain hidden sugars, preservatives, and additives that are not conducive to the Carnivore Diet. It's important to become familiar with reading labels and understanding what ingredients are acceptable on this eating plan.

Don't forget to check your spice rack as well. While many spices are allowed on the Carnivore Diet, some may contain fillers or anti-caking agents that are not compliant. Stick to pure, unadulterated spices to ensure you are staying on track with your diet.

Once you have cleared out your kitchen of non-compliant foods, it's time to restock with high-quality animal products such as grass-fed beef, pasture-raised poultry, wild-caught fish, eggs and organ meats (organ meats are not essential.) These nutrient-dense foods will be the foundation of your Carnivore Diet and will provide you with the essential nutrients your body needs to thrive.

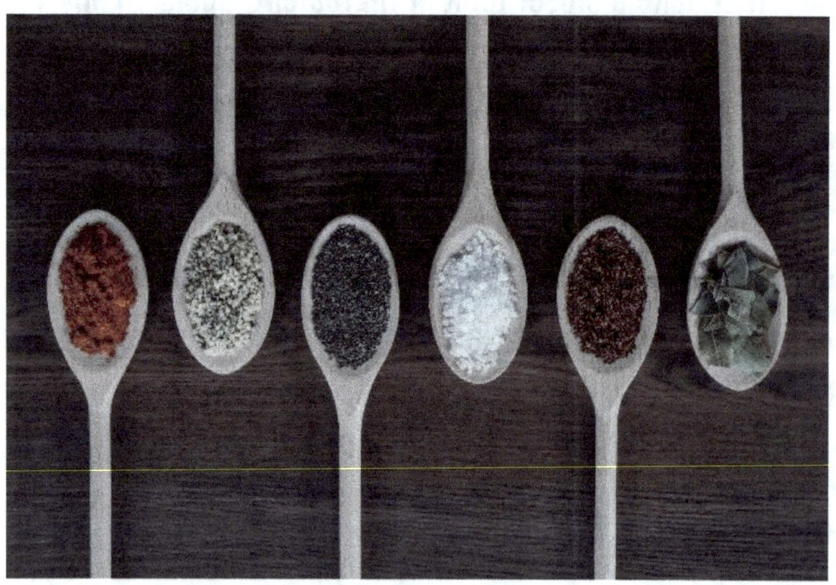

By taking the time to clear out your kitchen and restock with Carnivore-friendly foods, you are setting yourself up for success on this transformative journey to better health and body composition. Embrace this opportunity to make positive changes in your life and enjoy the benefits of the Carnivore Diet.

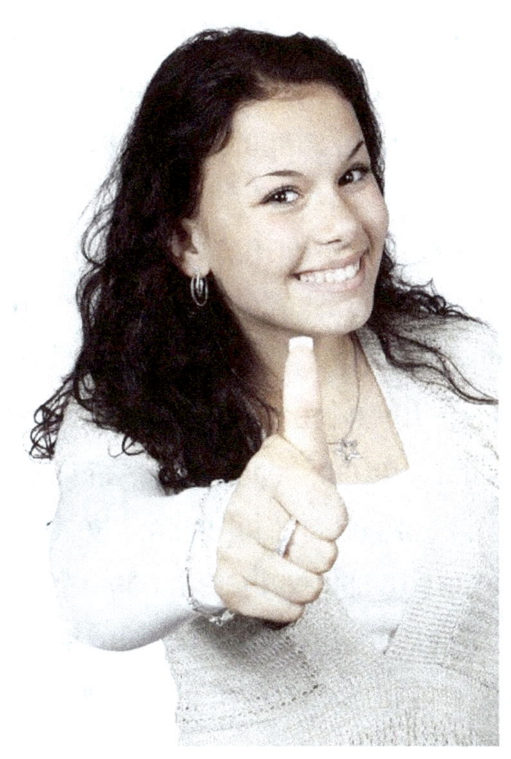

Stocking Up on Carnivore-Friendly Foods

When starting the carnivore diet, it is essential to stock up on carnivore-friendly foods to ensure a successful transition and optimize your health and body composition. In this subchapter, we will discuss the key foods you should include in your pantry and fridge to support your carnivore lifestyle.

First and foremost, prioritize high-quality animal products such as grass-fed beef, pastured poultry, wild-caught fish, eggs and organ meats if you like organ meats. These foods are rich in essential nutrients like protein, healthy fats, and vitamins and minerals that are crucial for overall health and well-being. Be sure to source these foods from reputable suppliers to ensure they are free from antibiotics, hormones, and other harmful additives.

In addition to animal products, consider stocking up on other carnivore-friendly foods like bone broth, and high-fat dairy products like butter and cheese (raw if possible.) These foods provide additional nutrients and variety to your diet while still aligning with the principles of the carnivore diet.

When selecting carnivore-friendly foods, focus on nutrient density and quality rather than quantity. It's important to prioritize foods that are rich in essential nutrients and free from inflammatory compounds like grains, legumes, and processed foods that are not part of the carnivore diet.

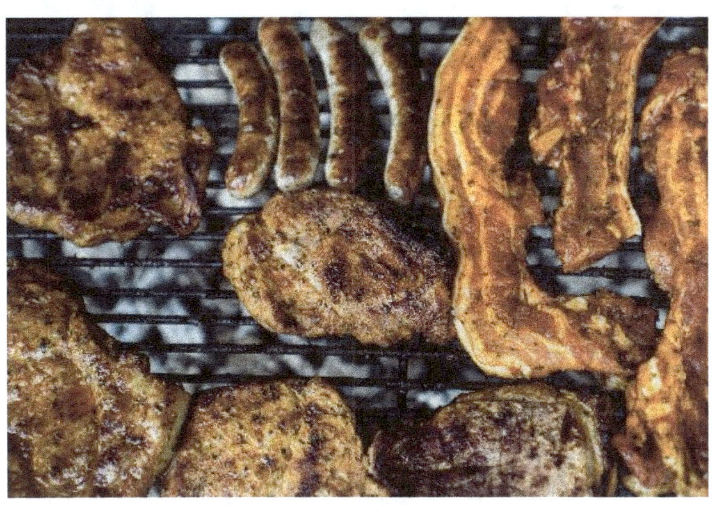

By stocking up on carnivore-friendly foods, you can set yourself up for success on the carnivore diet and optimize your health and body composition. With a well-stocked pantry and fridge, you can easily prepare delicious and nutritious meals that support your goals and help you thrive on the carnivore lifestyle.

There is a handy shopping list builder on my website
https://www.theukcarnivore.com/interactive-tools/shopping-list

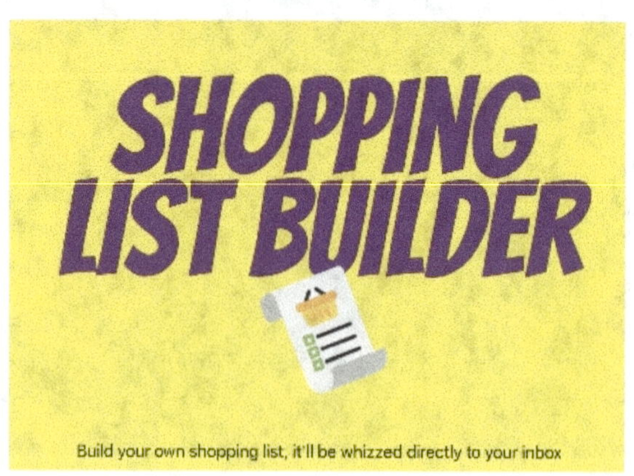

Chapter 3: Transitioning to the Carnivore Diet

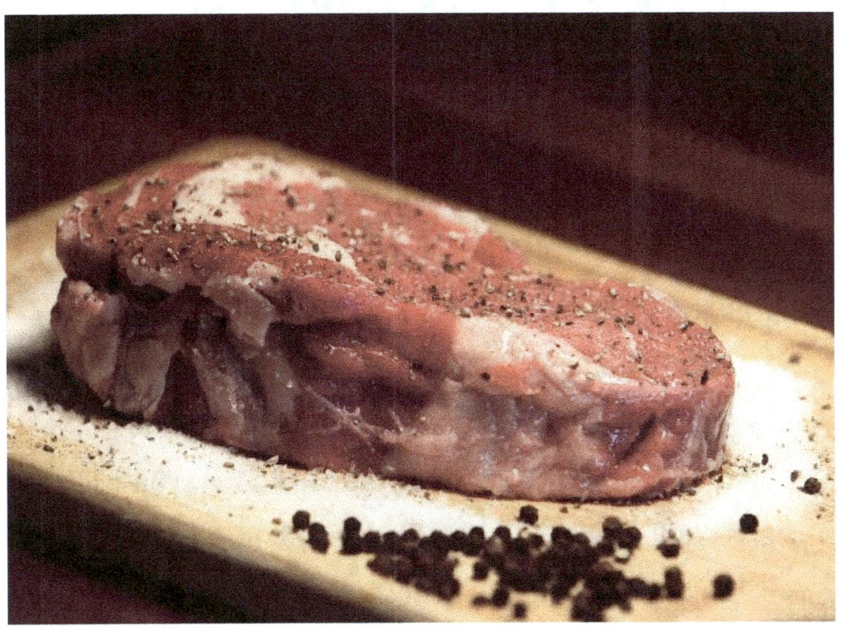

Gradual Transition or Cold Turkey Approach

When it comes to adopting the carnivore diet, one of the biggest decisions you'll have to make is how you want to approach the transition from your current eating habits. There are two main schools of thought on this topic: the gradual transition approach and the cold turkey approach.

The gradual transition approach involves slowly eliminating non-carnivorous foods from your diet over a period of time. This can be helpful for people who are used to eating a wide variety of foods and are worried about feeling deprived or overwhelmed by a sudden change. By gradually reducing the amount of non-carnivorous foods you eat, you can give your body time to adjust to the new way of eating without experiencing severe withdrawal symptoms.

On the other hand, the cold turkey approach involves cutting out all non-carnivorous foods from your diet all at once. While this approach can be more challenging initially, it can also lead to faster results and a quicker adaptation to the carnivore diet. Some people find that going cold turkey helps them commit fully to the new way of eating and prevents them from slipping back into old habits.

Ultimately, the decision of whether to take a gradual transition or cold turkey approach to the carnivore diet comes down to personal preference and what you think will work best for you. Experiment with both methods and see which one helps you achieve your health and body composition goals most effectively. Remember, the most important thing is to listen to your body and make choices that support your overall well-being.

Study: Plant Toxins

The factors behind the development of leaky gut are still under active research, but various foods contain compounds that have been linked to increased intestinal permeability.

These gut-harming compounds and the foods that contain them warrant further consideration. Plants employ chemical defenses, such as plant toxins and antinutrients, in their efforts to survive and reproduce.

When humans consume these plant-based foods, these defense mechanisms come into contact with our gut lining. Plant toxins and antinutrients play a significant role in intestinal permeability, as frequent low-dose exposure to these compounds can contribute to leaky gut.

Although most cultivated plant foods are not immediately toxic, continual low-dose exposure can lead to leaky gut. Common plant compounds known to contribute to leaky gut include oxalates, histamines, phytic acid, lectins, and carbohydrates.

Additionally, a notable proportion of grains, spices, and dried fruits may be contaminated with bacteria and mycotoxins (toxic molds), which have also been implicated in intestinal permeability.

https://www.tandfonline.com/doi/full/10.1080/23311932.2016.1191103

https://www.ncbi.nlm.nih.gov/pmc/articles/PMC8744955/

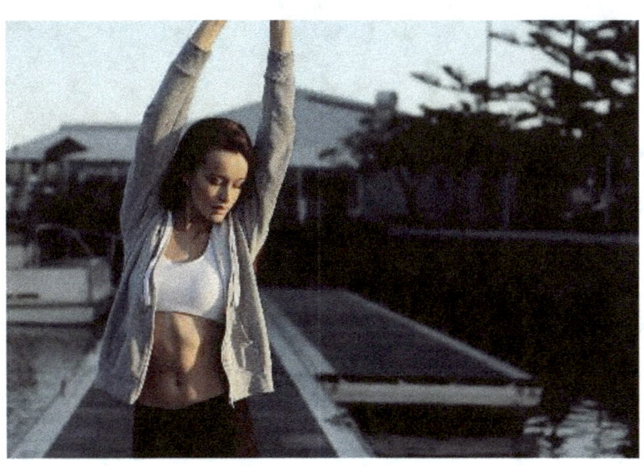

Dealing with Withdrawal Symptoms

When starting the carnivore diet, it's common to experience withdrawal symptoms as your body adjusts to the new way of eating. These symptoms can be uncomfortable, but they are a sign that your body is detoxing and adapting to the elimination of certain foods from your diet.

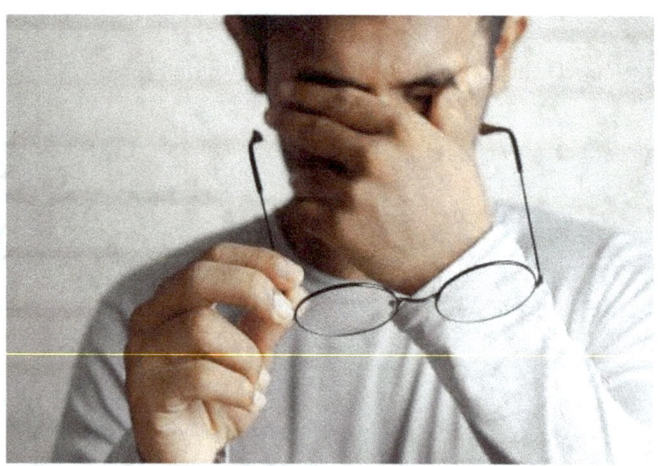

One of the most common withdrawal symptoms when starting the carnivore diet is the "keto flu." This is a collection of symptoms that can include fatigue, headaches, irritability, and nausea. These symptoms typically last for a few days to a week as your body transitions from burning carbohydrates for fuel to burning fat.

To help alleviate these symptoms, it's important to stay hydrated and consume electrolytes. Drinking plenty of **water with electrolytes** and adding salt to your meals can help replenish the electrolytes that your body may be losing during the transition period.

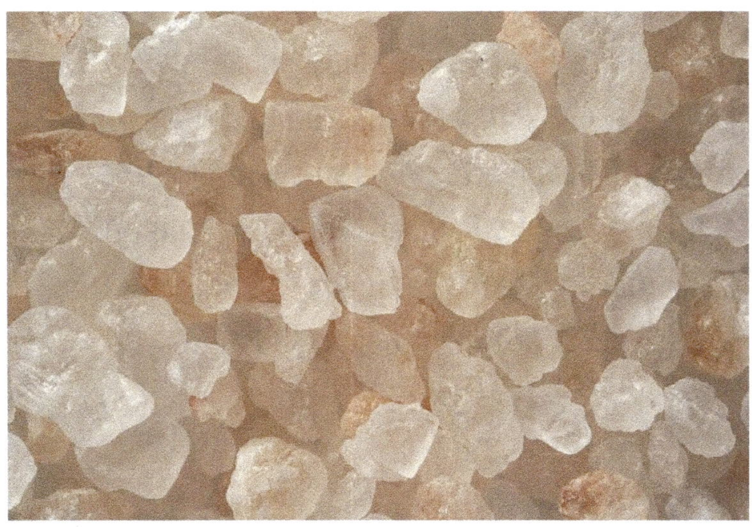

Another common withdrawal symptom when starting the carnivore diet is cravings for sugar and carbohydrates. These cravings can be intense, but they will diminish over time as your body adjusts to the new way of eating. To help combat these cravings, focus on eating plenty of protein and healthy fats to keep you satiated and satisfied.

It's also important to be patient with yourself during this transition period. Remember that your body is going through a significant change, and it may take time to fully adapt to the carnivore diet. Be kind to yourself and give yourself grace as you navigate these withdrawal symptoms.

By staying hydrated, consuming electrolytes, and being patient with yourself, you can effectively deal with withdrawal symptoms when starting the carnivore diet. Remember that these symptoms are temporary and are a sign that your body is healing and adapting to a healthier way of eating.

Common Challenges and How to Overcome Them

Starting the Carnivore Diet can be an exciting journey towards better health and body composition. However, like any new dietary approach, it comes with its own set of challenges. In this subchapter, we will explore some of the common challenges that people face when starting the Carnivore Diet and provide practical tips on how to overcome them.

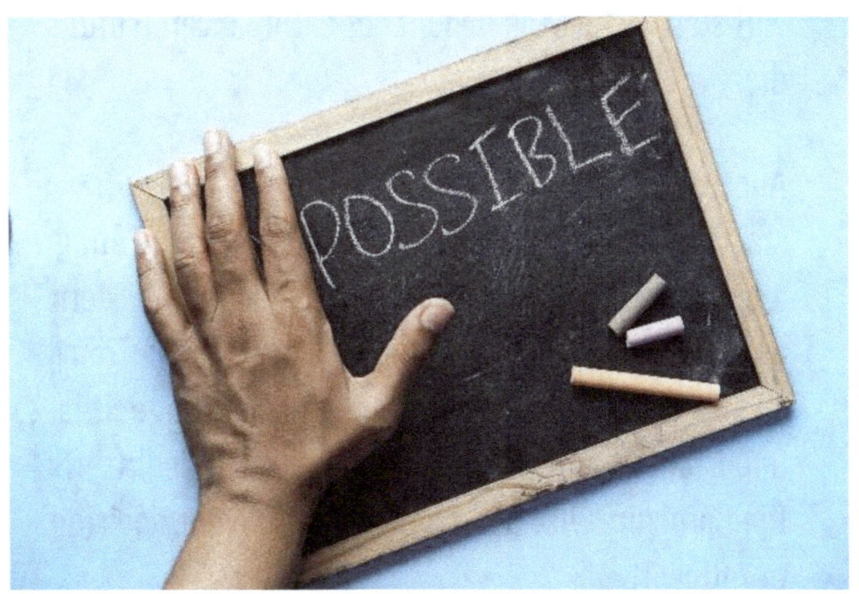

One of the most common challenges when starting the Carnivore Diet is the initial adjustment period. Your body may take some time to adapt to this new way of eating, especially if you are coming from a diet high in carbohydrates. During this period, you may experience symptoms such as fatigue, headaches, and cravings as your body detoxes from sugar and other non-carnivorous foods. To overcome this challenge, it is important to stay hydrated, get plenty of rest, and be patient with yourself. Your body will eventually adapt to the new diet, and you will start to feel the benefits of eating a carnivorous diet.

Another challenge that many people face when starting the Carnivore Diet is social pressure. Eating a diet that is so different from the standard Western diet can be met with skepticism and criticism from friends and family. To overcome this challenge, it is important to educate yourself about the benefits of the Carnivore Diet and be confident in your decision to follow it.

Surround yourself with like-minded individuals who support your dietary choices and focus on the positive changes you are experiencing in your health and body composition.

By being aware of these common challenges and implementing the tips provided, you can successfully navigate the transition to the Carnivore Diet and reap the many benefits it has to offer. Remember, consistency is key, and with time and patience, you will achieve your health and body composition goals.

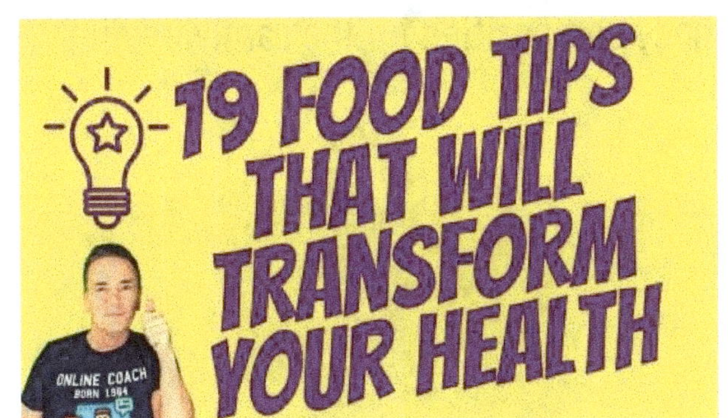

Help is never far away on my YouTube channel
https://youtu.be/KUArRWlmXec

Chapter 4: Optimizing Your Carnivore Diet

Balancing Macronutrients

Balancing macronutrients is a crucial aspect of the carnivore diet. Macronutrients are the three main components of our diet: protein, fats, and carbohydrates. Understanding how to balance these macronutrients is key to achieving optimal health and body composition on the carnivore diet.

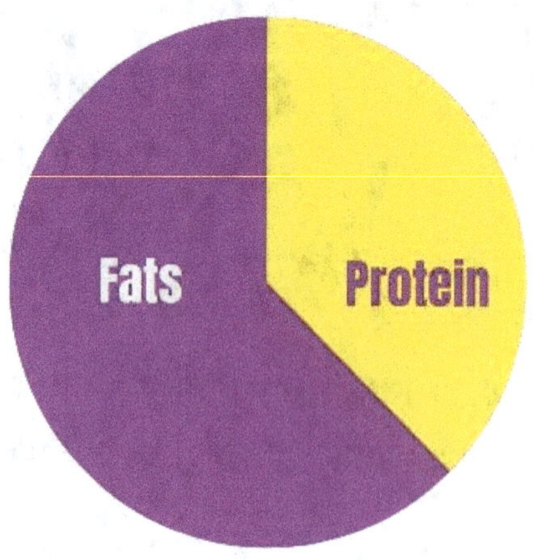

Protein could be seen as the foundation of the carnivore diet, as it provides essential amino acids that our bodies need to function properly. Aim to include high-quality sources of protein such as beef, pork, poultry, eggs and fish in your meals. Protein should be a priority in regards as to eating enough of it as it builds structures in your body, repairs tissue, maintains muscles, maintains bones and is helpful in many other processes.

Fats are also an important macronutrient on the carnivore diet, as they provide a concentrated source of energy and help to keep you feeling full and satisfied. Include healthy sources of fats such as butter, ghee, tallow, and lard in your meals to ensure you are getting enough of this essential nutrient. Eating fatty 'cuts' of meats can be really delicious and beneficial. When buying ground beef (called mince in the UK) you can look for 80/20, which means 80% protein and 20% fat. Eggs are a fabulous source of healthy fat.

Carbohydrates are not a focus on the carnivore diet, as it is a low-carb way of eating. However, some individuals may find that including small amounts of carbohydrates from sources like dairy or organ meats can be beneficial for their overall health and well-being.

To balance your macronutrients on the carnivore diet, aim to prioritize protein while including healthy fats and minimal carbohydrates in your meals. Experiment with different ratios of macronutrients to find what works best for your body and goals.

By understanding and balancing your macronutrients on the carnivore diet, you can optimize your health and body composition while enjoying delicious and satisfying meals. Remember that everyone is different, so listen to your body and make adjustments as needed to find what works best for you.

How much to eat?

How Much To Eat? **The simple answer is to eat as much as it takes to feel full.** Meat is an incredible filler, and you'll be surprised how little it will take to keep you going for many hours while on the carnivore diet.

The general rules
Protein:
1gram of protein per pound of your lean bodyweight (if you weigh 170lbs you need 170 grams of protein, simple)
Fat:
1gram of fat per pound of your lean bodyweight.
As above, it's that simple to start. Then it becomes a matter of trial and error as some thrive with higher fat while others do really well on lean protein.

Another example
You want to weigh 100lb then you need 100 grams of protein and 100 grams of fat.
This is around 66% fat and 34% protein by 'calories.' As you adapt to this way of eating, you might need more or less. How can you tell? Your body will tell you! If you start to gain unwanted body fat you may need to eat less fat.

One big caveat here, if you are healing then this is normal and many people gain a little body fat but feel so much healthier. Once the healing has taken place then the body composition starts to improve. Some people can eat up to 2.5lbs of meat per day, other folk do well on less.

For example a very fit carnivore I know eats around 300-350g per day spread over 2 meals and he weighs 175lbs. Dr Shawn Baker mentioned on the Joe Rogan #1050 podcast interview how he has seen many people eat on average about 2 lbs (900 grams) of meat per day.

What To Eat (Meats)

Red Meat: Pork, Beef, Lamb, and Game

White Meat: Turkey, Chicken, Fish, and Seafood

Organ Meat: Liver, Kidney, Bone Marrow, Heart

For the majority of people, these will provide all the nutrition you need, including vitamins, minerals, and protein.

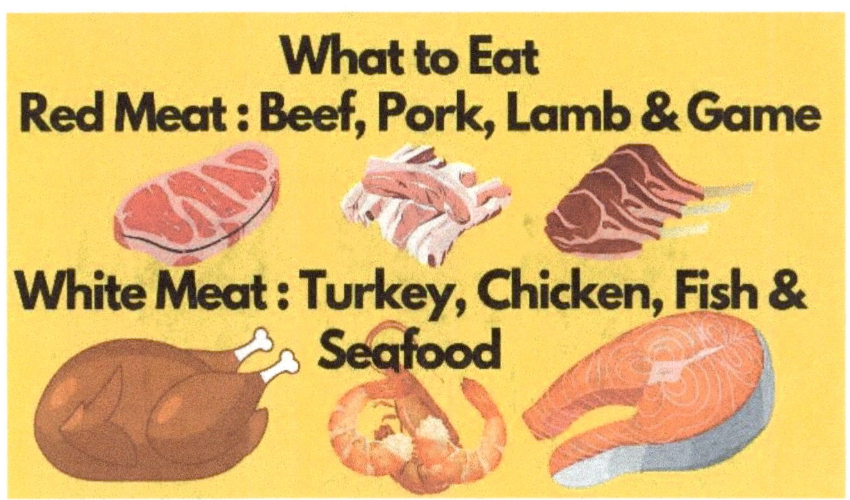

What To Eat (Eggs and Dairy)

Eggs: Chicken, Duck, and Goose Eggs

Dairy: Butter, Cheese, and Cream

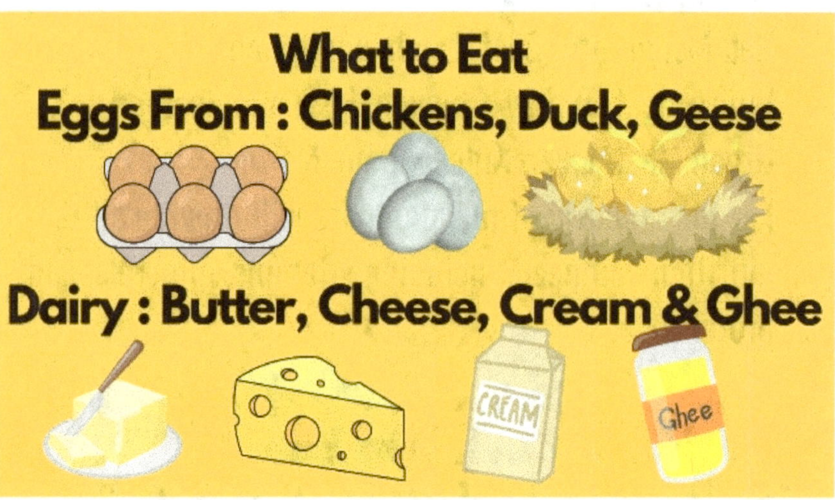

**Workouts on the
Carnivore Experience App**

Incorporating Organ Meats and Seafood

Incorporating organ meats and seafood into your carnivore diet can provide a wide range of health benefits and help you achieve better body composition. Organ meats, such as liver, heart, and kidneys, are incredibly nutrient-dense and packed with essential vitamins and minerals. Seafood, on the other hand, is an excellent source of omega-3 fatty acids, which are crucial for brain health, reducing inflammation, and supporting overall well-being. Sardines are a great source of calcium. **Organ meats are NOT ESSENTIAL but are an OPTION.**

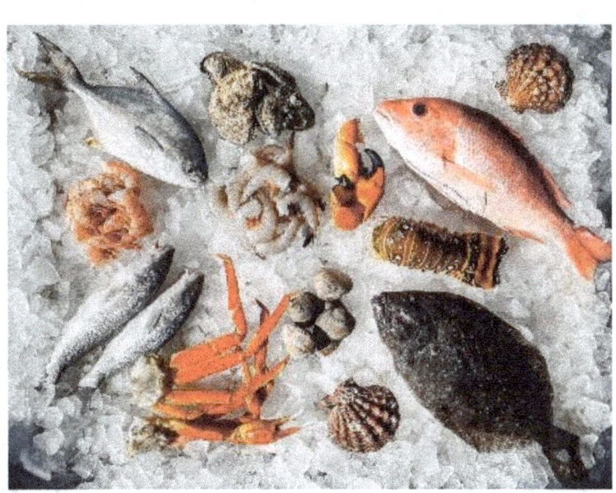

The Carnivore Experience

When starting the carnivore diet, it's important to include a variety of animal-based foods to ensure you're getting all the nutrients your body needs. Some people believe that organ meats are particularly beneficial, as they contain high amounts of vitamin A, B vitamins, iron, and zinc. Incorporating these nutrient-dense foods into your diet can help improve your energy levels, support your immune system, and promote optimal organ function. Experience in this field has shown that organ meats are not an essential part of this way of eating.

Seafood is another important component that can bring you to a well-rounded carnivore diet. Fish, shrimp, and other seafood options are rich in omega-3 fatty acids, which have been shown to reduce inflammation, improve heart health, and support brain function. Including seafood in your diet can help balance out the omega-6 fatty acids found in other foods, leading to a healthier ratio of omega-3 to omega-6 fats in your body.

By incorporating organ meats and seafood into your carnivore diet, you may be able to take your health and body composition to the next level. These nutrient-dense foods provide essential vitamins, minerals, and fatty acids that are crucial for optimal health and well-being. Experiment with different cuts of meat, organs, and seafood options to find what works best for you and enjoy the benefits of a well-rounded carnivore diet.

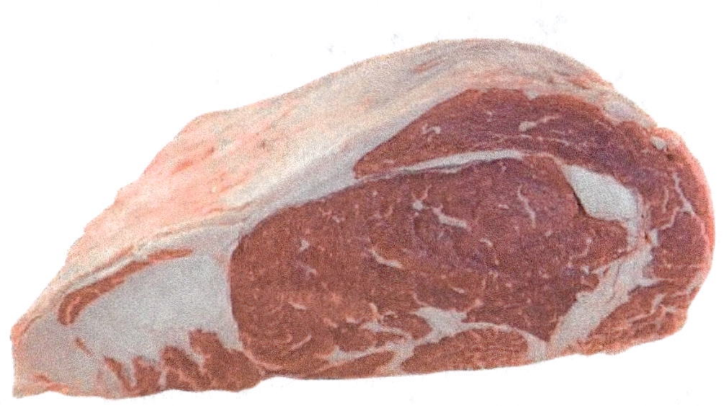

Understanding the Importance of Quality Meat

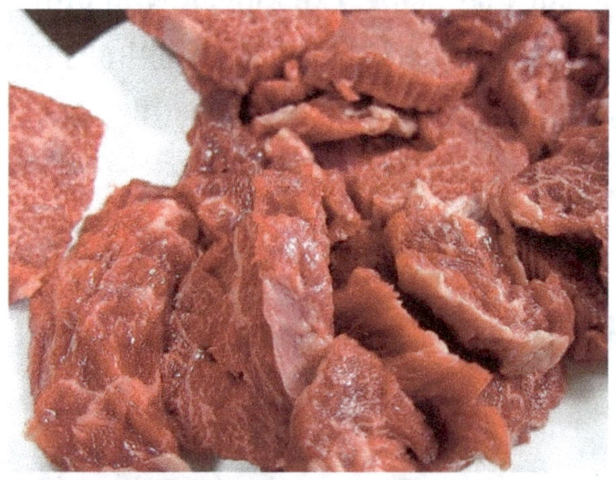

Understanding the importance of quality meat is essential when starting the Carnivore Diet. High-quality meat is packed with essential nutrients like protein, vitamins, and minerals that are crucial for overall health and well-being. When you consume high-quality meat, you are providing your body with the building blocks it needs to function optimally.

One of the key benefits of quality meat is its protein content. Protein is essential for muscle growth, repair, and maintenance. By including quality meat in your diet, you can ensure that your body has an adequate supply of protein to support your fitness and health goals.

Quality meat is also a rich source of important vitamins and minerals like iron, zinc, and B vitamins. These nutrients play a vital role in various bodily functions, including energy production, immune function, and hormone regulation. By choosing quality meat, you can ensure that you are getting a wide range of essential nutrients to support your overall health.

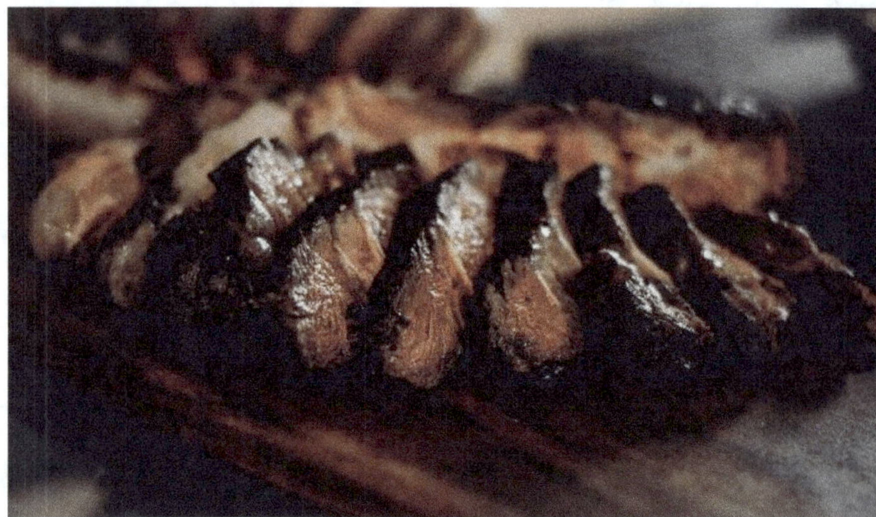

In addition to its nutritional benefits, quality meat should be free from harmful additives, preservatives, and artificial ingredients that are often found in processed meats.

By opting for high-quality, unprocessed meat, you can avoid potentially harmful substances and ensure that you are consuming a clean, natural source of nutrition.

Overall, understanding the importance of quality meat is crucial for anyone looking to improve their health and body composition. By including high-quality meat in your diet, you can provide your body with the nutrients it needs to thrive and reach your health and fitness goals on the Carnivore Diet.

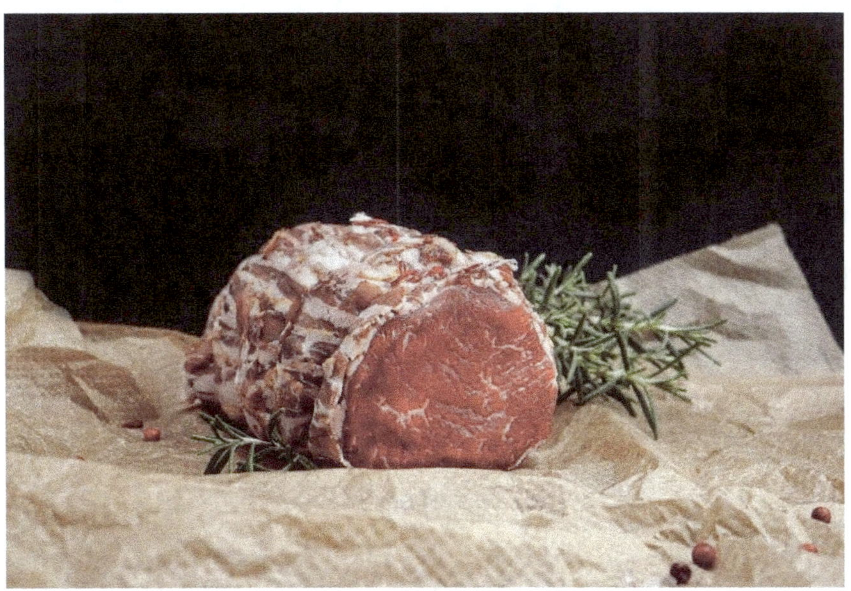

What To Drink?

Water (just drinking water is optimal.)
Flat is generally better than sparkling if you suffer with belching)
Coffee (Swiss Water Decaf, I recommend avoiding caffeine for fat loss)
Tea, including herbal teas, are OK Drinks as long as you don't sweeten them with any type of sugar.

What you want to avoid is any type of drink that contains carbs like sodas, fruit and veg juices, and energy drinks as these will disrupt your fat loss if that is your goal.

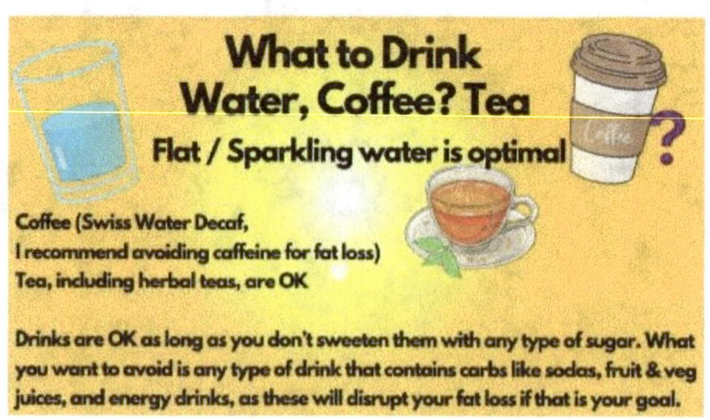

Chapter 5: Fine-Tuning Your Carnivore Diet

Tracking Your Progress

Once you have made the decision to start the Carnivore Diet, tracking your progress is essential to ensure you are on the right path to achieving your health and body composition goals. But this way of eating is different.

You can track by just assessing how you look and feel. Noticing how well your clothes fit compared to when you started for example. These types of things are tracking. But some people need more concrete proof. Although I do not recommend this detailed way of tracking your way of eating and progress, in some cases the need to track is strong.

Keeping track of your food intake, weight, and any changes in your body can help you make adjustments to your diet and lifestyle as needed. You need to have patience as it may be a few weeks before changes are easily apparent, while you may be getting healthier in the background even in the very early stages.

One of the most common ways to track your progress on the Carnivore Diet is by keeping a food and mood journal. This can help you identify any patterns in your eating habits, as well as any foods that may be causing you issues. By writing down everything you eat and how you feel after eating, you can begin to see how different foods affect your body.

In addition to keeping a food and mood journal, **tracking your weight and body measurements can also be helpful in monitoring your progress. Again this is something I do not recommend but some people just have to do it!**

Standing on a scale can help you see if you are losing weight, gaining muscle, or making other changes to your body composition. Remember that weight fluctuations are normal, so it is important to focus on long-term trends rather than day-to-day changes. But please be aware of what are known as 'non-scale-victories,' such as better sleep, more energy, better hair, less anxiety and other benefits of this kind

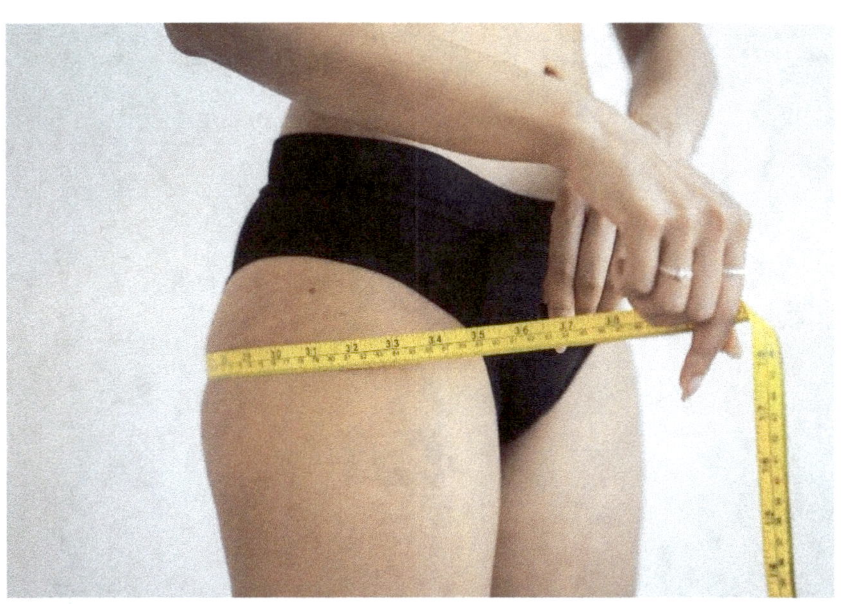

I would say that the most important aspect of tracking your progress on the Carnivore Diet is paying attention to how you feel. Are you experiencing **more energy, better digestion, more sleep or improved mental clarity?** These are all positive signs that you are on the right track. If you are experiencing negative symptoms, such as fatigue or digestive issues, it may be a sign that you need to make adjustments to your diet.

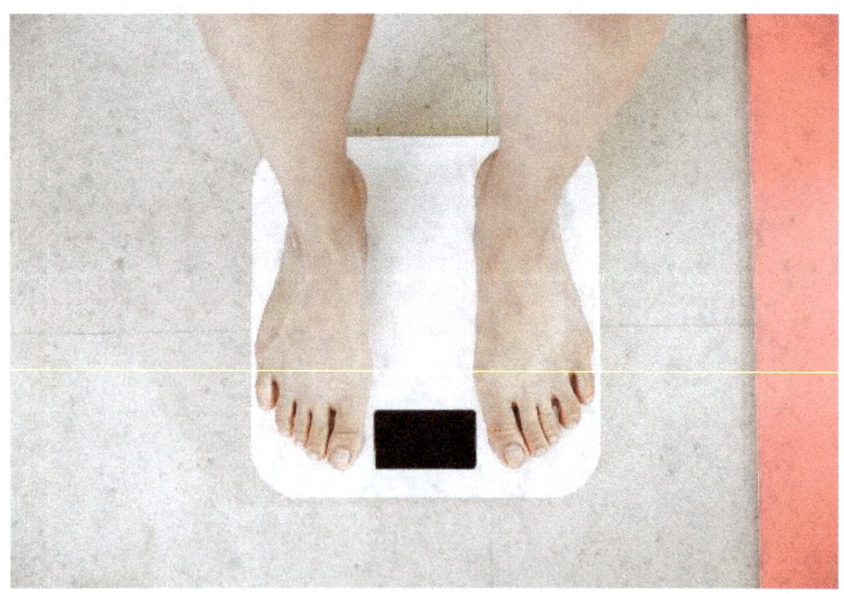

Overall, tracking your progress on the Carnivore Diet can help you stay motivated and make informed decisions about your health and body composition. By paying attention to what you eat, how you feel, and any changes in your body, you can ensure that you are on the path to better health. On the next page there is a simple check list to write down some of your goals.

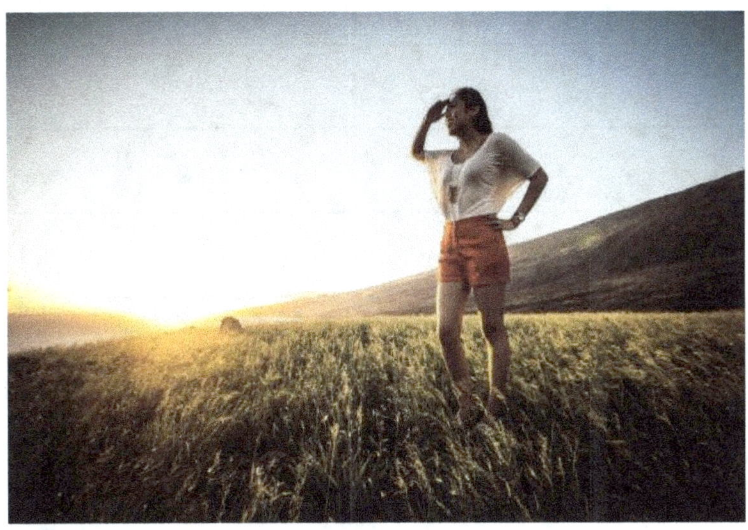

To do list

Start to plan your goals based on the tips you learned

In 6 months from now I want to achieve...

☐ ____

☐ ____

☐ ____

☐ ____

☐ ____

Making Adjustments Based on Your Goals

Once you have started the Carnivore Diet and have begun to see the positive changes in your health and body composition, it's important to continue making adjustments based on your goals. Whether you are looking to lose weight, improve your athletic performance, or simply feel better overall, tailoring your Carnivore Diet to meet your specific needs is key to long-term success.

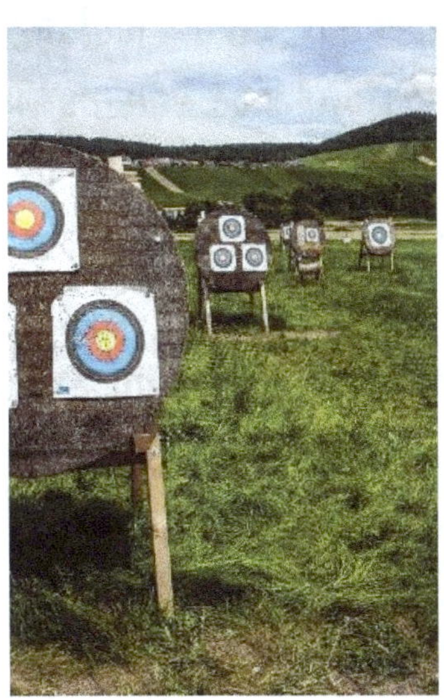

If your goal is the loss of body fat, you may need to adjust your portion sizes or meal frequency or remove things like dairy, which can stall some people. While the Carnivore Diet is naturally satiating, it's still possible to overeat if you are not mindful of your satiety signals. Keeping track of your food intake and monitoring your progress can help ensure you are on the right track to reaching your weight loss goals.

On the other hand, if you are looking to improve your athletic performance, you may need to experiment with adding more fats or protein to your meals to support your energy needs. Some athletes find that increasing their intake of fatty cuts of meat or incorporating more organ meats into their diet helps them perform at their best.

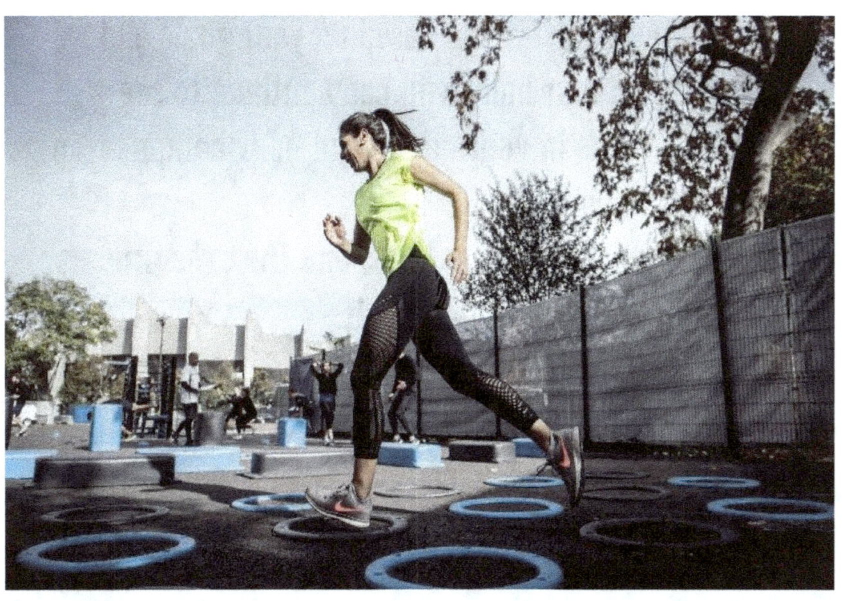

Ultimately, listening to your body and making adjustments based on how you feel is crucial to achieving your goals on the Carnivore Diet. Pay attention to how certain foods make you feel and adjust your intake accordingly. Remember, the Carnivore Diet is not a one-size-fits-all approach, so don't be afraid to experiment and find what works best for you.

By making adjustments based on your goals and listening to your body, you can continue to see improvements in your health and body composition on the Carnivore Diet.
Stay committed to your goals and trust the process your body will thank you for it.

Try my online commitment builder
https://www.theukcarnivore.com/interactive-tools/commitment-builder

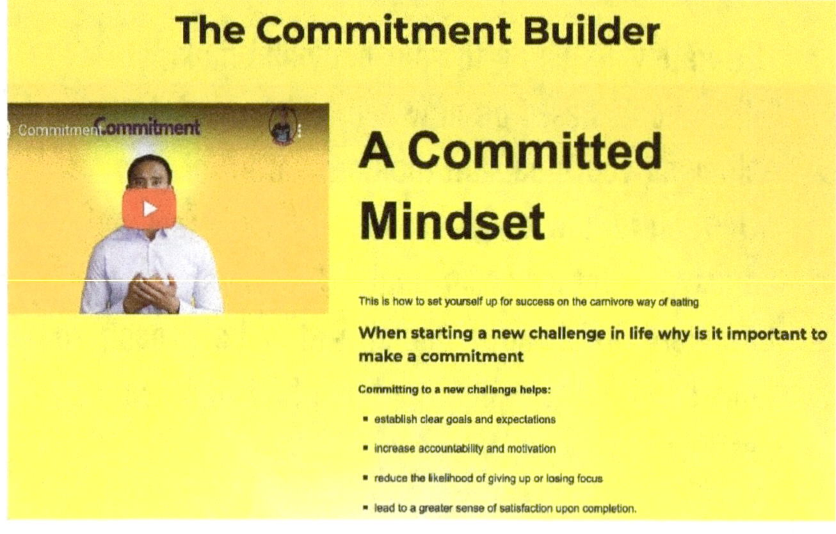

Listening to Your Body's Signals

One of the key components of successfully starting the Carnivore Diet is learning to tune in to your body's signals. Our bodies are incredibly intelligent and are constantly sending us messages about what they need to function optimally. By paying attention to these signals, you can better understand what your body is trying to tell you and make adjustments to your diet and lifestyle accordingly.

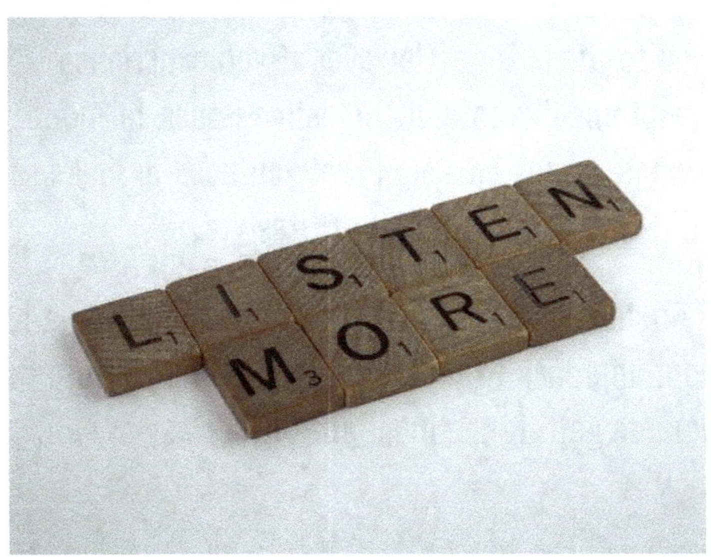

When you first start the Carnivore Diet, it's essential to listen to how your body responds to the changes you are making. Pay attention to things like your energy levels, digestion, mood, and overall well-being. These are all important indicators of how your body is reacting to the new way of eating.

If you notice that you are feeling more energized, focused, and satisfied on the Carnivore Diet, these are all positive signs that your body is responding well to the change. However, if you experience symptoms like fatigue, digestive issues, or mood swings, it may be a sign that you need to make some adjustments to your diet or lifestyle.

By listening to your body's signals, you can fine-tune your approach to the Carnivore Diet and ensure that you are getting the most out of this way of eating.

Remember that everyone's body is different, so what works for one person may not work for another. By paying attention to how your body responds and making adjustments as needed, you can set yourself up for success on the Carnivore Diet and improve your overall health and body composition.

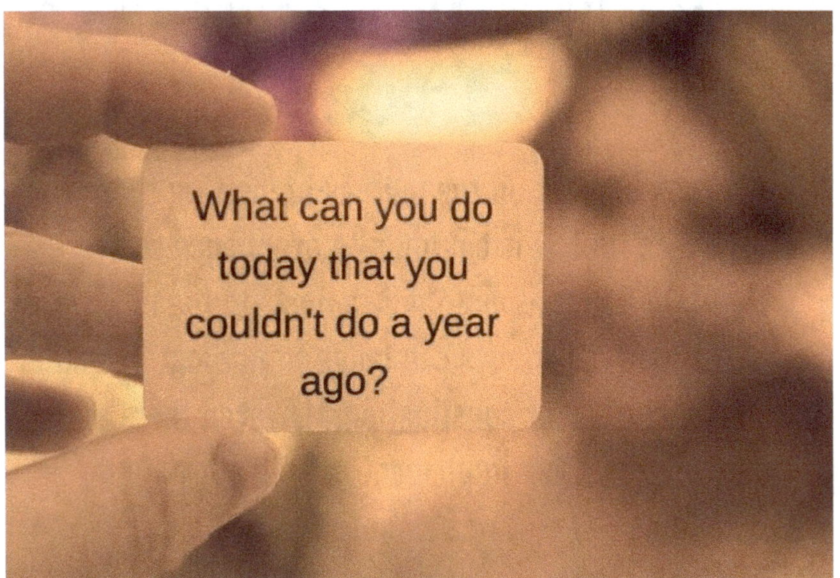

Chapter 6: Troubleshooting Common Issues

Dealing with Digestive Issues

When embarking on the journey of starting the Carnivore Diet, it is common to experience some digestive issues as your body adjusts to the new way of eating. These issues can range from bloating and gas to diarrhea or constipation. However, there are strategies you can implement to help alleviate these symptoms and ensure a smooth transition to the Carnivore Diet.

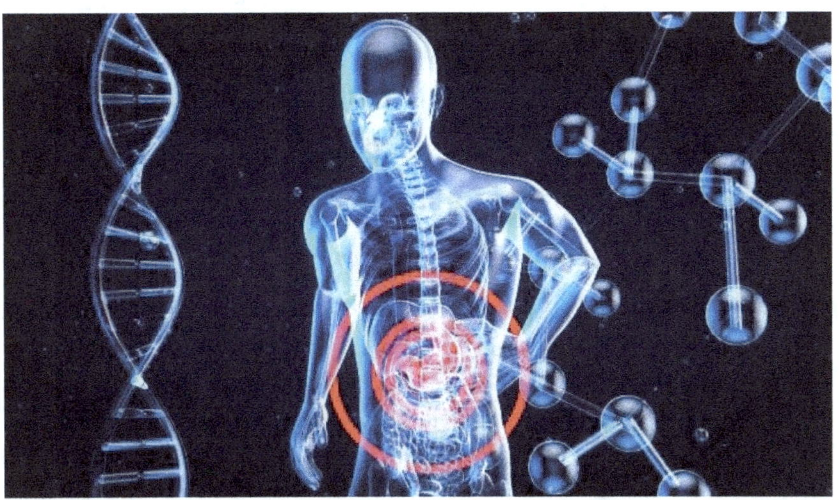

One of the most important things to remember when dealing with digestive issues is to give your body time to adapt. The sudden shift from a diet high in carbohydrates and fiber to one that is primarily meat-based can be a shock to your digestive system. Be patient with your body and allow it time to adjust to the new way of eating.

Another key factor in dealing with digestive issues on the Carnivore Diet is to focus on the quality of the meat you are consuming. Opt for grass-fed, organic meats whenever possible, as they are higher in nutrients and free from harmful chemicals and additives that can exacerbate digestive issues. Additionally, be mindful of how you are preparing your meat – avoid overcooking, as this can make it harder for your body to digest.

Incorporating bone broth into your daily routine can also be beneficial for soothing digestive issues on the Carnivore Diet. Bone broth is rich in collagen and gelatin, which can help repair the lining of your gut and improve digestion. Sipping on a warm cup of bone broth before meals can help prepare your stomach for the incoming meat.

Lastly, stay hydrated and make sure you are getting enough electrolytes, especially in the initial stages of starting the Carnivore Diet. Proper hydration is essential for healthy digestion, and electrolytes can help maintain the balance of fluids in your body.

By implementing these strategies and being patient with your body, you can effectively deal with digestive issues and set yourself up for success on the Carnivore Diet. Remember, everyone's body is different, so it's important to listen to your body and adjust your approach as needed.

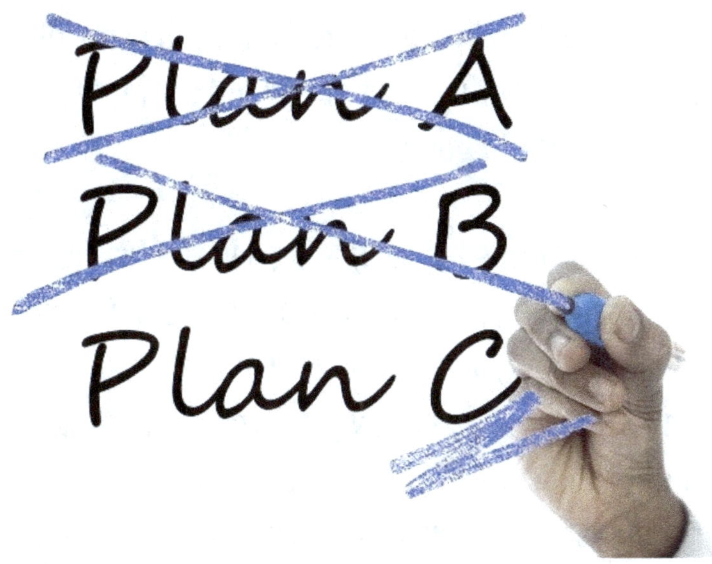

Handling Social Situations and Eating Out

Handling Social Situations and Eating Out can be a challenge when following the Carnivore Diet, but with some preparation and strategies, you can still enjoy social gatherings and dining out while staying true to your health goals.

One of the key tips for navigating social situations is to communicate your dietary needs and preferences to friends, family, and restaurant staff in advance. Letting others know about your Carnivore Diet can help them understand your choices and make accommodations for you. This can also prevent any awkward situations or misunderstandings when it comes to meal options.

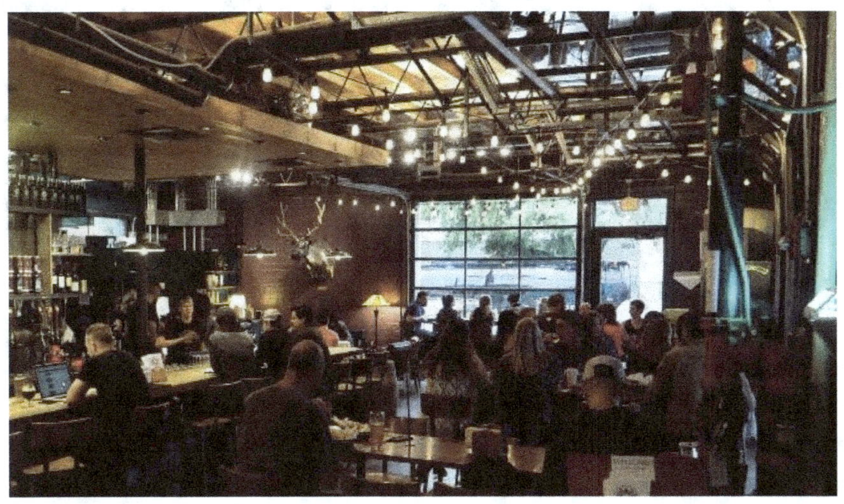

When dining out, look for steak houses, barbecue joints, or seafood restaurants that offer a variety of meat options. You can also customize your order by asking for simple preparations like grilled or broiled meats without sauces or seasonings. Many restaurants are willing to accommodate special requests, so don't be afraid to ask for what you need.

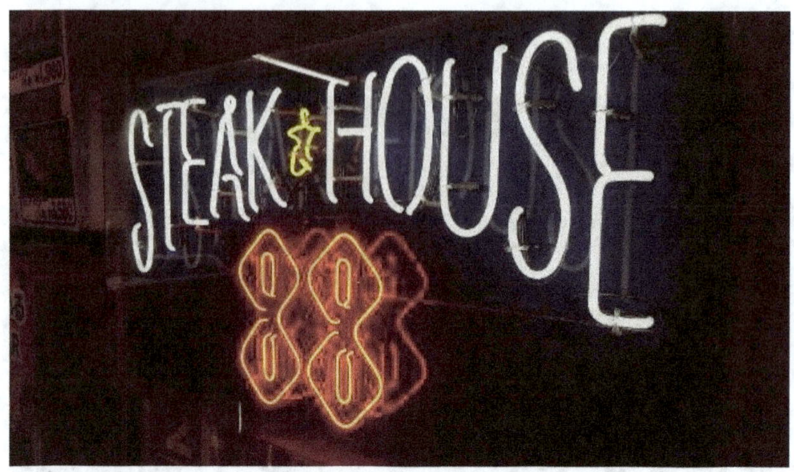

If you're attending a social gathering or potluck, consider bringing your own dish to share. This way, you can ensure there will be something for you to eat that aligns with your Carnivore Diet. Grilled meats, charcuterie boards, or deviled eggs are great options that are both delicious and Carnivore-friendly.

Remember that it's okay to politely decline food that doesn't fit your dietary plan. Focus on enjoying the company and conversation rather than feeling pressured to eat something that doesn't align with your goals. By being prepared and proactive, you can navigate social situations and eating out while staying on track with your Carnivore Diet journey.

Accusations of Nutrient Deficiencies

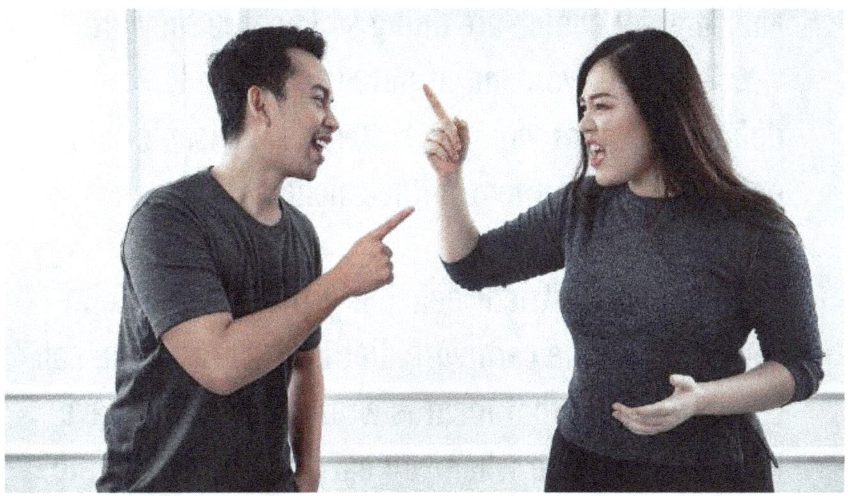

When embarking on the carnivore diet, it's crucial to address any potential nutrient deficiency questions that may arise due to the misrepresented nature of this way of eating.

While the carnivore diet is actually rich in animal proteins, nutrients, vitamins, minerals and essential fats, many people wrongly believe that it may lack certain essential vitamins and minerals that they inaccurately believe are abundant in plant-based foods.

It's important to be mindful that people questioning your dietary choice are doing so because they are worried about you and of potential nutrient deficiencies that you may suffer. It's advisable to be polite and guide them to the science.

One common nutrient deficiency that people claim can occur on the carnivore diet is vitamin C. You can educate people that meat is wrongly stated to have no vitamin C, also when you eat a low carbohydrate diet your body needs much less vitamin C to perform optimally. Some carnivore diet followers still have some doubts and they often consider incorporating organ meats like liver, which are high in vitamin C, or taking a vitamin C supplement to meet their daily requirements.

Another potential deficiency that people tell you to watch out for is fiber, as the carnivore way of eating eliminates all plant-based sources of fiber.

There are many articles that show fiber is not needed in a species specific diet. Again some carnivore followers worry about this aspect initially and to prevent constipation and promote gut health, individuals on the carnivore diet can consume bone broth.

Additionally, micronutrients like magnesium, potassium, and calcium may also be CLAIMED to be lacking in a carnivore way of eating. But there are no deficiencies, individuals can consume foods like fatty cuts of meat, fatty fish, eggs, and dairy products, which are rich in these essential minerals.

By being proactive about addressing potential accusations of nutrient deficiencies on the carnivore way of eating, individuals can optimize their health and body composition while reaping the benefits of this unique way of eating without anyone making them feel unsure about what they are doing. With careful planning and attention to their dietary needs, those looking to improve their health and body composition can successfully navigate the carnivore diet and achieve their wellness goals.

Chapter 7: Sustaining Your Carnivore Lifestyle

Creating a Long-Term Plan

Creating a long-term plan is essential when embarking on the journey of starting the Carnivore Diet. This plan will not only help you stay on track but also ensure that you are making sustainable changes to your health and body composition.

One of the first steps in creating a long-term plan is setting realistic goals. Whether your goal is to lose weight, improve your energy levels, stabilise your blood sugar or simply feel better overall, it's important to have a clear vision of what you want to achieve.

By setting specific, measurable, attainable, relevant, and time-bound (SMART) goals, you can track your progress and stay motivated throughout your Carnivore Diet journey. In the Carnivore Experience App there are 30-day and 60-day plans to follow with daily guidance and more in-depth information about everything mentioned in this book.

Another key aspect of a long-term plan is meal planning. Planning your meals in advance can help you stay on track with your diet and make healthier choices. By stocking your kitchen with Carnivore-friendly foods and preparing meals ahead of time, you can avoid the temptation of reaching for unhealthy snacks or fast food when hunger strikes. There is a meal plan on the website and in the app.

Additionally, it's important to listen to your body and make adjustments to your plan as needed. Everyone is different, and what works for one person may not work for another.

Pay attention to how your body responds to the Carnivore Diet and make changes accordingly. This could involve adjusting your macronutrient ratios, incorporating intermittent fasting, or experimenting with different types of meat.

By creating a long-term plan for your Carnivore Diet journey, you can set yourself up for success and achieve your health and body composition goals. Stay committed, stay consistent, and remember that progress takes time. With dedication and perseverance, you can experience the many benefits of the Carnivore Diet and transform your health for the better.

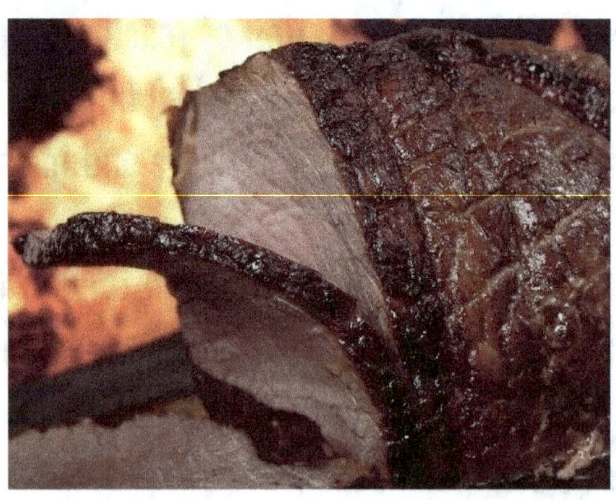

Staying Motivated and Focused

Embarking on a new diet can be both exciting and challenging. As you begin your journey on the carnivore diet, it's important to stay motivated and focused on your goals. Here are some tips to help you stay on track and make the most of your carnivore diet experience.

First and foremost, it's essential to set clear and realistic goals for yourself. Whether you're looking to improve your health, lose weight, or increase your energy levels, having a clear vision of what you want to achieve will help keep you motivated throughout your carnivore diet journey. Write down your goals and revisit them regularly to stay focused on your progress.

Another key to staying motivated on the carnivore diet is to stay informed and educated about the benefits of this way of eating. Understanding the science behind the carnivore diet and how it can positively impact your health and body composition can help reinforce your commitment to this lifestyle.

Additionally, finding a supportive community of like-minded individuals can provide you with the encouragement and motivation you need to stay on track. Join online forums, social media groups, or local meetups to connect with others who are also following the carnivore diet. Sharing your experiences, challenges, and successes with others can help keep you motivated and accountable.

Lastly, don't forget to celebrate your wins, no matter how small they may seem. Recognize and reward yourself for sticking to your carnivore diet plan, making healthy choices, and achieving your goals. By acknowledging your progress and staying positive, you'll be more likely to stay motivated and focused on your journey to better health and body composition.

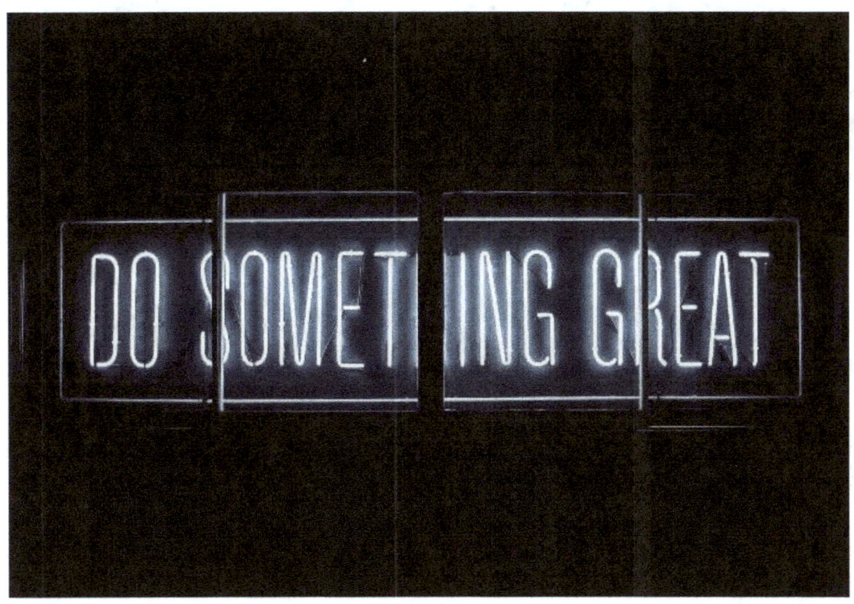

Remember, staying motivated and focused on the carnivore diet is a journey, not a destination. Keep pushing forward, stay committed to your goals, and you'll soon reap the benefits of this transformative way of eating.

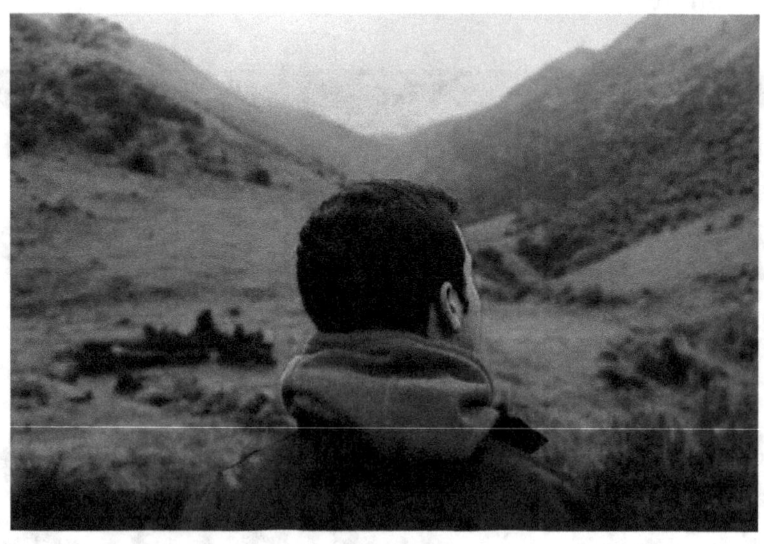

Celebrating Your Successes

As you embark on your journey to better health and body composition through the Carnivore Diet, it is important to take the time to acknowledge and celebrate your successes along the way. Whether it's shedding those extra pounds, improving your energy levels, or seeing a reduction in inflammation, every small victory is a step in the right direction towards achieving your ultimate health goals.

One way to celebrate your successes is by setting small, achievable goals for yourself and tracking your progress. For example, you could aim to incorporate more grass-fed meats into your diet, or commit to getting a certain number of hours of quality sleep each night. By setting specific goals and regularly monitoring your progress, you will be able to see how far you've come and feel a sense of accomplishment with each milestone you reach.

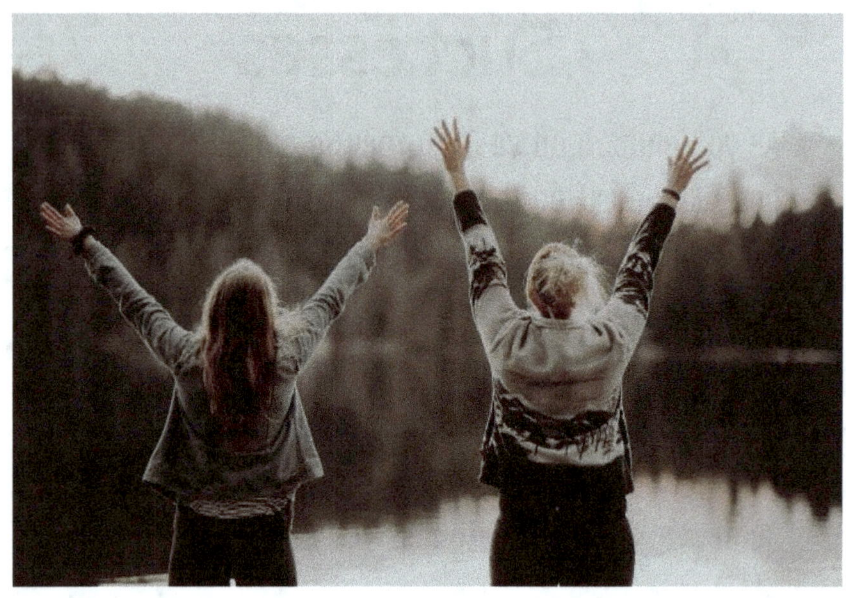

Another way to celebrate your successes is by rewarding yourself for your hard work. Treat yourself to a new piece of workout gear, a relaxing massage, or a delicious steak dinner as a way to acknowledge your dedication to your health journey. By rewarding yourself for your efforts, you will be more motivated to continue making positive choices for your well-being.

Remember, celebrating your successes is an important part of maintaining your momentum and staying committed to your health goals. By acknowledging your achievements, setting new goals, and rewarding yourself along the way, you will be better equipped to stay on track and continue making progress towards a healthier, happier you. Let each success be a reminder of how far you've come and how much more you are capable of achieving on your Carnivore Diet journey.

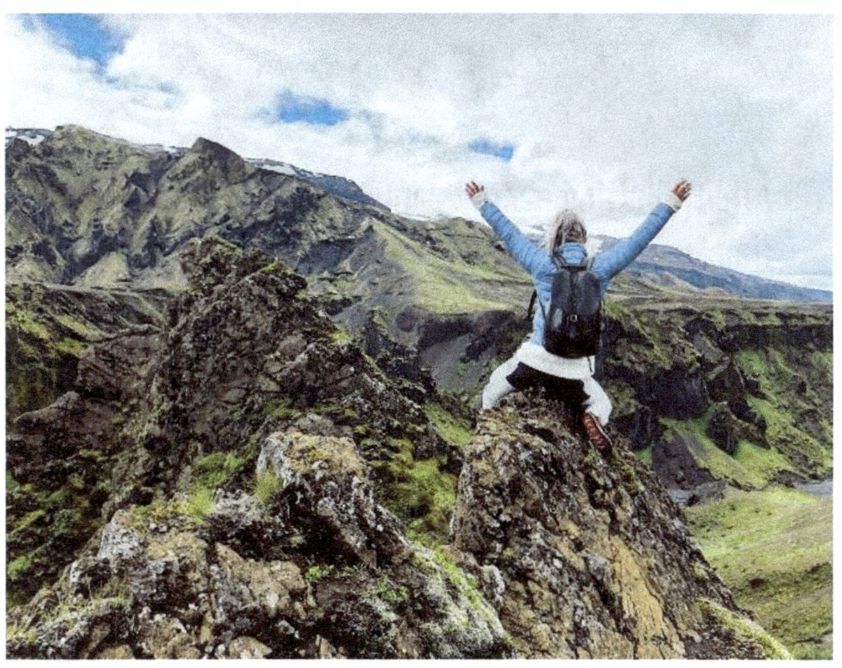

Chapter 8: Beyond the Carnivore Diet

Reintroducing Foods After a Period of Carnivore Eating

After following a strict carnivore diet for a period of time, you may be wondering how to reintroduce other foods back into your diet. I simply ask, "why would you do that?"

The foods that made you sick or overweight or both have no place in your way of life. Foods that made you anxious or lose sleep don't need to be reintroduced.

The carnivore way of eating is also a way of life. I have many success stories of long-term carnivores. Some have followed this way of eating for over 40 years, some for 30, 20 or a decade. I am in my fifth year of this way of eating and do not miss any of the foods that made me pre-diabetic, have a CAC of 639, lower left quadrant pain, perpetual athlete's foot and sun sensitivity.

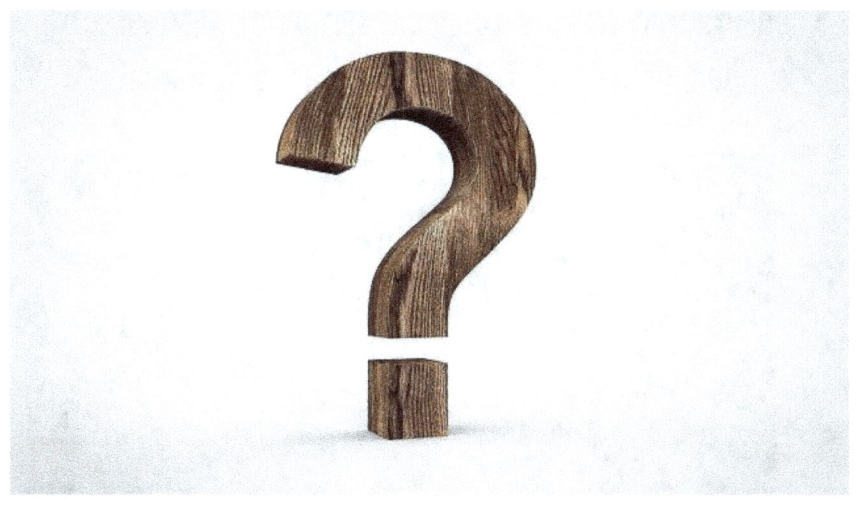

Finding Balance in Your Diet

Finding balance in your diet is crucial when embarking on any new eating plan, including the Carnivore Diet. While the focus of this diet is on consuming animal-based foods, it's important to ensure that you are getting a variety of nutrients to support your health and body composition goals.

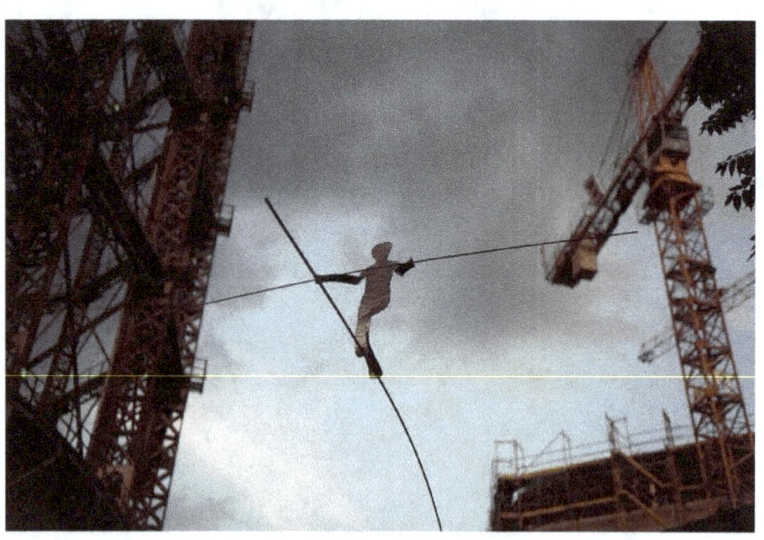

One way to achieve balance on the Carnivore Diet is by incorporating a variety of animal-based foods into your meals. This includes different types of meat, such as beef, chicken, pork, and fish, as well as organ meats like liver and heart. Each type of meat offers a unique set of nutrients that can help you meet your body's needs.

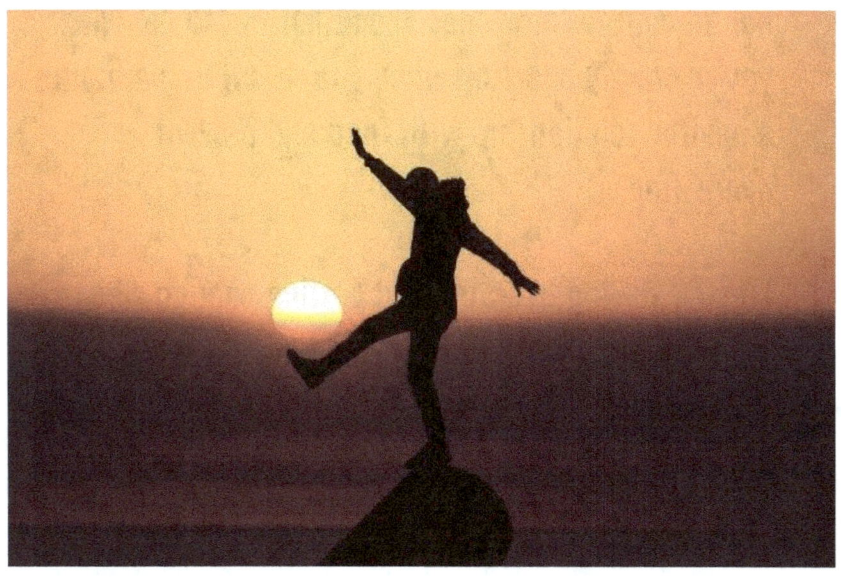

In addition to meat, it's important to include other sources of nutrients in your diet, such as eggs and dairy products if you tolerate them. These foods provide essential vitamins and minerals that may be lacking in a meat-only diet.

Another key aspect of finding balance on the Carnivore Diet is paying attention to your body's hunger and fullness cues. **It's important to eat when you're hungry and stop when you're full** to maintain a healthy relationship with food and prevent overeating.

Finally, staying hydrated and getting enough sleep are also important factors in achieving balance on the Carnivore Diet. Proper hydration supports digestion and overall health, while adequate sleep is crucial for recovery and optimal body composition.

By finding balance in your diet on the Carnivore Diet, you can support your health and body composition goals while enjoying the many benefits this eating plan has to offer. Remember to listen to your body, incorporate a variety of animal-based foods, and prioritize hydration and sleep for optimal results.

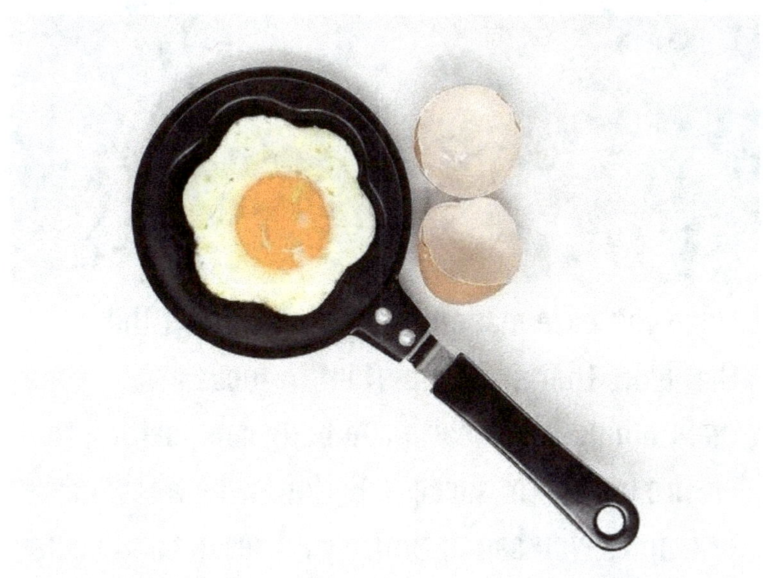

Maintaining Your Health and Body Composition

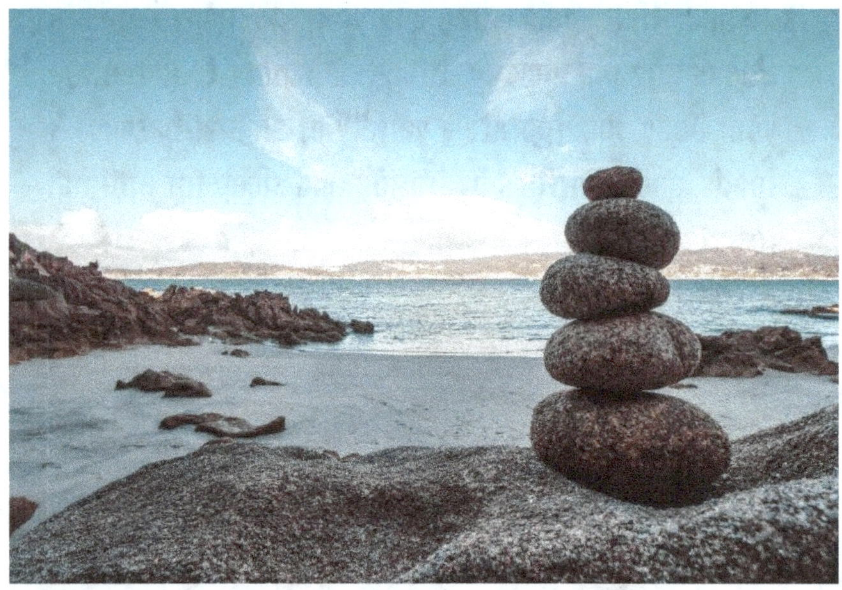

Once you have made the decision to start the Carnivore Diet, it is important to focus on maintaining your health and body composition to ensure long-term success. By following a few key principles, you can optimize your results and achieve your health goals.

One of the most important aspects of maintaining your health and body composition on the Carnivore Diet is to prioritize nutrient-dense foods. This means focusing on high-quality animal products such as grass-fed beef, wild-caught fish, and pastured eggs. These foods are rich in essential nutrients like protein, vitamins, and minerals that are crucial for overall health and well-being.

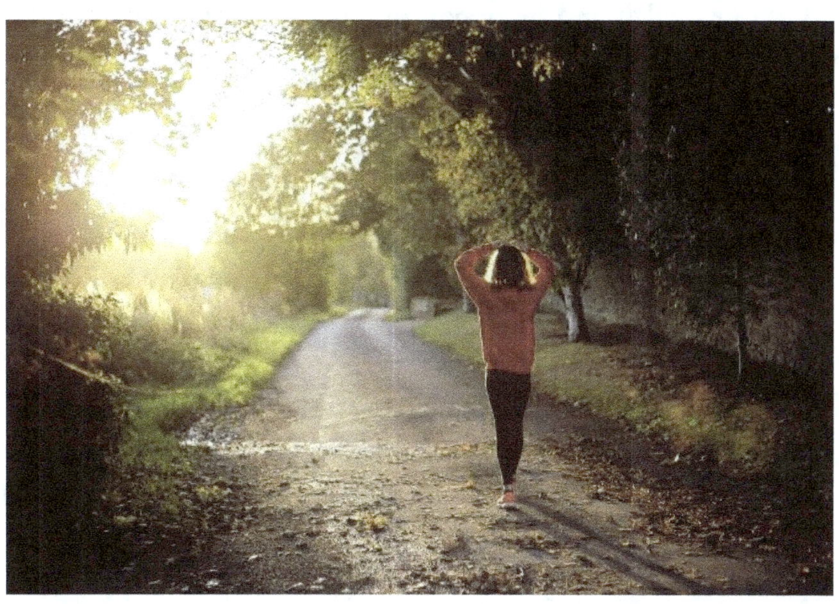

In addition to eating nutrient-dense foods, it is important to pay attention to portion sizes and meal timing. While the Carnivore Diet is known for its emphasis on satiety, it is still possible to overeat and hinder your progress. Be mindful of your hunger cues and stop eating when you feel satisfied.

Regular physical activity is also key to maintaining your health and body composition on the Carnivore Diet. Incorporating strength training into your routine can help you build lean muscle mass, improve your metabolism, and support overall health.

Lastly, it is important to listen to your body and make adjustments as needed. If you are not seeing the results you desire, consider consulting with a specialist to help tailor the Carnivore Diet to your individual needs.

Study: Leaky Gut

Leaky Gut.

New research indicates that sugar-rich diets, such as the Standard American Diet, have been linked to the increased dominance of bacteria associated with intestinal permeability, namely Proteobacteria.

Simultaneously, these high-sugar diets have been found to reduce the prevalence of gut-protective Bacteroidetes, which are crucial for reinforcing gut barrier function and battling endotoxins.

https://www.ncbi.nlm.nih.gov/pmc/articles/PMC7284805/

Additional studies have revealed that high-sugar diets can compromise the integrity of the intestinal barrier, ultimately prompting systemic autoimmune responses.

https://pubmed.ncbi.nlm.nih.gov/25288760/

Moreover, insufficient levels of beneficial gut bacteria, a condition referred to as gut dysbiosis, may yield similar outcomes.

For mitigating the impact of sugar on leaky gut, it is advisable to eliminate added sugars and high-carb foods, including candy, soda, baked goods such as cookies, cakes, and pastries, bread products, and high-carb vegetables and fruits.

https://www.ncbi.nlm.nih.gov/pmc/articles/PMC7766268/

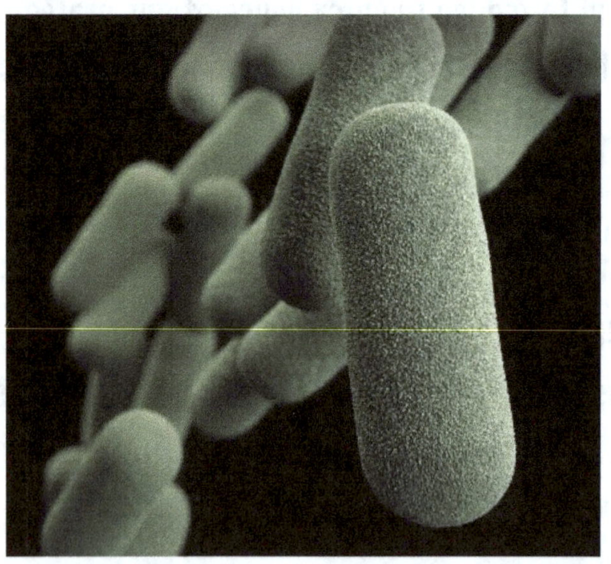

Your Carnivore Experience To Better Health

By following these principles and staying committed to your health goals, you can maintain your health and body composition on the Carnivore Diet for the long term. Remember, consistency is key, and small changes over time can lead to significant improvements in your overall health and well-being.

In conclusion, this Carnivore Diet Blueprint offers a comprehensive roadmap for those looking to improve their health and body composition through a carnivorous lifestyle. By following the guidelines outlined in this book, you will be able to optimize your nutrient intake, enhance your energy levels, and achieve your fitness goals.

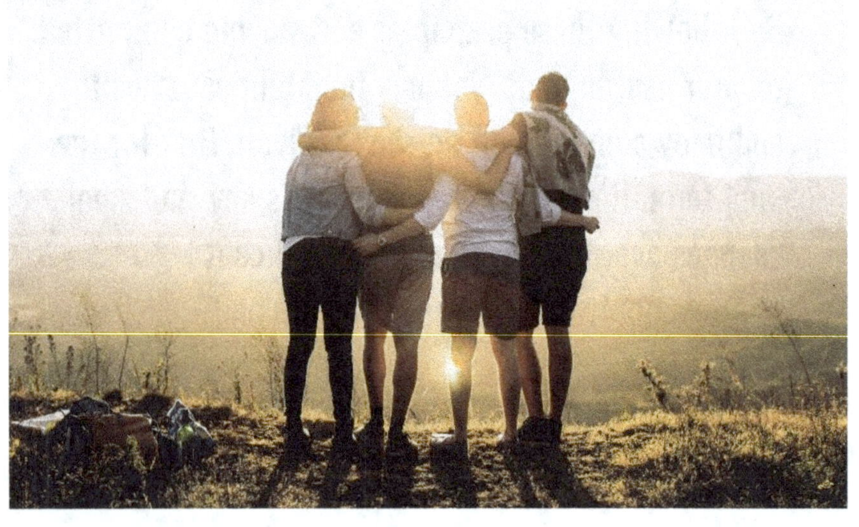

It is important to remember that **the Carnivore Diet is not a one-size-fits-all approach.** It is essential to listen to your body and make adjustments as needed. Pay attention to how different foods make you feel and adjust your diet accordingly.

As you embark on your carnivorous journey, remember to prioritize high-quality, nutrient-dense animal products. Opt for grass-fed, organic meats whenever possible, and vary your protein sources to ensure a well-rounded nutrient profile.

Additionally, be mindful of your hydration and electrolyte levels, as these are crucial for optimal health and performance on the Carnivore Diet. Consider incorporating bone broth, salt, and other electrolyte-rich foods into your daily routine to support your body's needs.

Feel free to write down any after-reading insights
and thoughts

Insights

Feel free to write down any after-reading insights and thoughts

In 6 months from now I want to achieve...

- ____

- ____

- ____

- ____

- ____

Insights

Finally, **remember that consistency is key.** Stay committed to your Carnivore Diet blueprint and give your body time to adapt to this new way of eating. With patience and dedication, you will begin to experience the many benefits of a carnivorous lifestyle, including improved energy, mental clarity, and body composition.

By following the guidelines outlined in this book, you are well on your way to better health and a stronger, leaner body. Embrace the Carnivore Diet blueprint and watch as your health and vitality soar to new heights.

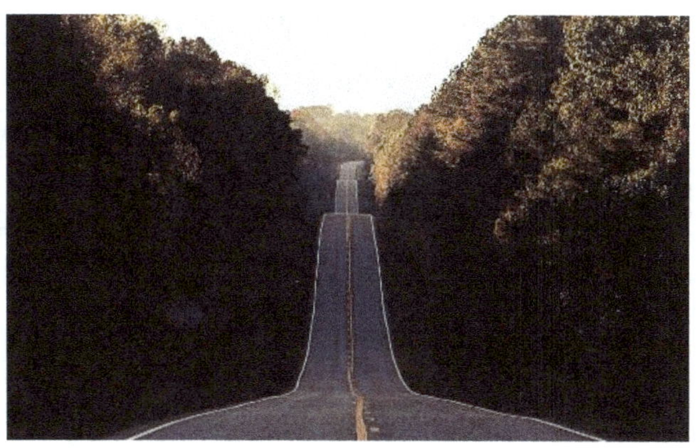

Summary

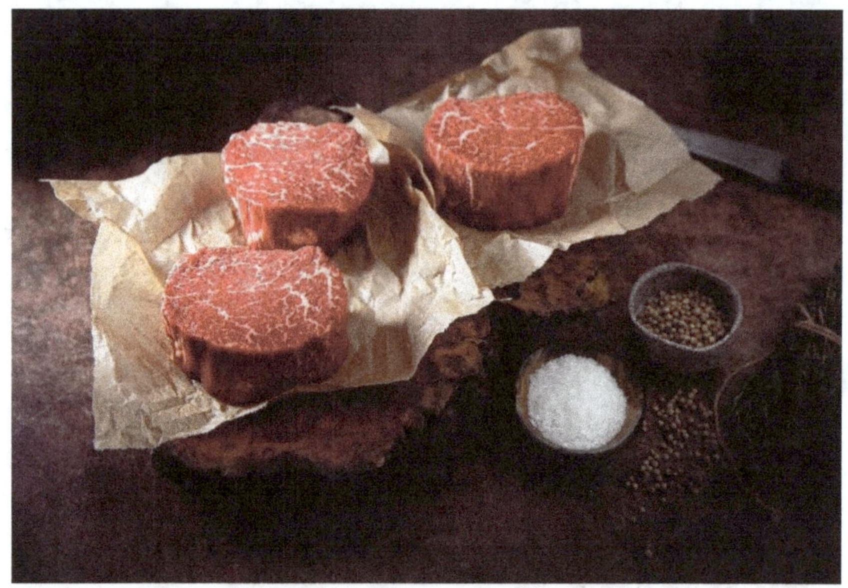

Feel free to write down any after-reading insights
and thoughts

**Next up is a little about my own personal experience
and then a section with the meal plan**

About The Author

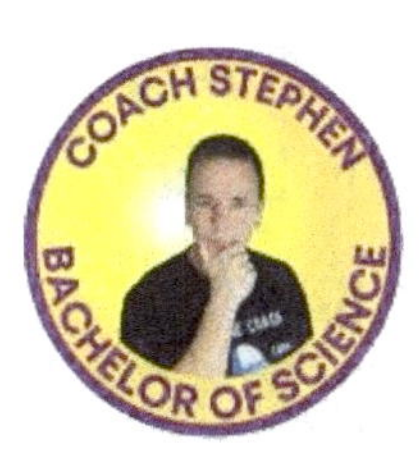

Hi, I'm Coach Stephen and in May 2024 I will be 60 years-old and at that point I will have been eating the carnivore way for 5 years. I hold a BSc.(Hons.) in physiology and health sciences. In the UK I obtained specialist practitioner status in managing Obesity and Diabetes (UK qualified) My interest in bio-hacking and lab tests was so strong that I trained to be a qualified phlebotomist, which means I am quite lucky in having access to blood work. Why do I tell you this?

So you can see that my main interest in my life is understanding how the human body works and applying that knowledge to help people either regain health or optimize those that are already reasonably fit.

At age 50 I tried low-carb and I did what most people do and I eventually tried Keto. The obvious progression from there was to try carnivore, it was by my 55th birthday. This was also when I studied under Dr Shawn Baker at MeatRx (now Revero) to become a certified online Coach. Currently I have over 1,000 reviews from happy clients from that platform and from the Steak and Butter Gang too.

Recently I began to document all the transformations in health and body composition and have a growing daily library of video success stories (over 130 at the time of writing) that I am immensely proud of and will be continually adding to.

I have had many health issues before going low-carb at age 50 By age 49 I was pre-diabetic, that has completely reversed. I had a coronary artery score of 639, but I am still alive after all these years! Lower left quadrant pain that required a colonoscopy investigating the issues. Resolved on Keto.

Deafness requires hearing aids, hearing has improved in the last 3 years! Which I have a YouTube video about. Skin rash on forehead, completely gone. Athlete's foot for over 30 years which I had not even realised had cleared up completely with no intervention, just nutrition. I was just so used to having it I'd forgotten all about it.

When I was 23 I was told by a very convincing doctor with images of my hip that I would be 'in a wheelchair by the time I was 50.' Well I got past 50 without that happening but I did have other issues going through my 30s and 40s. Rashes, colds, joint pains and knee trouble.

My digestion was a mess and I was very gassy (which also has thankfully gone) Plus I was getting tubbier and tubbier, even though I did not drink or smoke and I ate 'healthily' in inverted commas. Porridge, low-fat everything, freshly squeezed orange juice, grains, veggie and fruit etc.

Although my skin stretched from previously being overweight I got my abs back as well as my health thanks to carnivore and eating more! Possibly fasting will tighten up the skin over time? So all my 'health issues' have been resolved completely or managed to some degree.

At a very early age I started playing football and by the time I was 16 I was semi-professional. I still hold a Football Association coaching badge. I also have successfully coached an olympic athlete and in my forties I was a competitive runner and have competed in 5Km, 10Km, 10 mile and Half-Marathons.

Also coaching a 50-year-old overweight man to become one of the top 25% marathon runners in the world. I am enjoying my online coaching role, helping people achieve their goals, through exercise and low-carb, keto or a carnivore way of eating, making them feel fitter and better about themselves.

Some clients keep progressing and signing up for more, so that probably speaks volumes about how much they have got out of the online coaching or personal training experience.

It not always about training someone to be super fit, I get as much pleasure out of helping someone going from a Zimmer frame to walking or from having a very bent over back to being able to stand upright (see the before and after below)

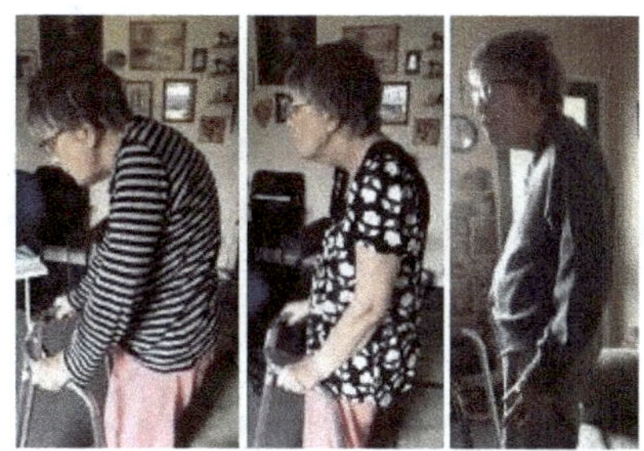

I have always enjoyed fitness and being around people that wish to push their body further, before qualifying as a Personal Trainer I competed in a Bodybuilding tournament and found plenty of people there going as far as they could push their body naturally.

Over the years I have tried lots of different 'healthy' eating styles and plans to help my training and to keep healthy, I have finally found one that makes perfect sense and works, this inspired me to write my own book.

I have also produced some health information videos for my community network and YouTube channel. I feel I am good at getting my point across and feel my workouts and videos are informative, fun and well presented.

This might owe something to my background in the media working as an actor, then as a stuntman in shows like Ultimate Force and finally as a body double in films such as Batman (The Dark Knight) and The Bourne Ultimatum.

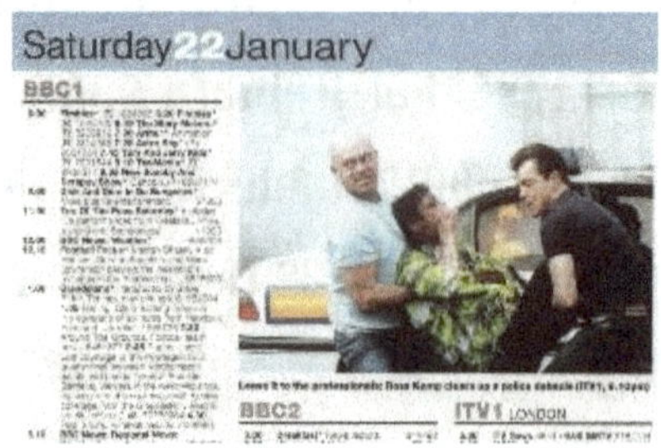

If you have a personal story you wish to share with me I would be glad to hear it.

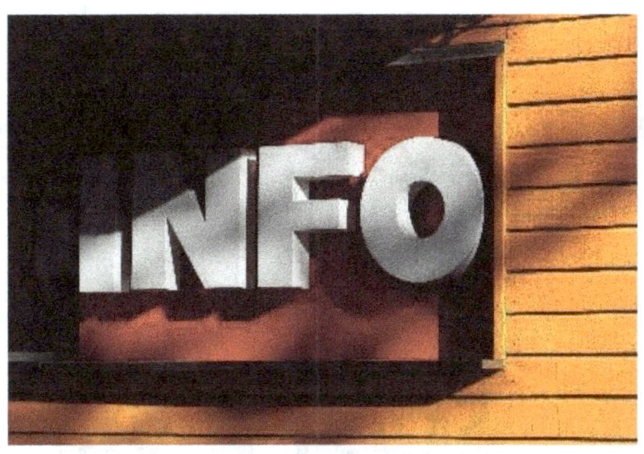

I am not a medical professional, and the information I provide is not intended as medical advice. I share my personal health experiences to help others, but it is important to seek guidance from a qualified healthcare professional regarding any health-related concerns or questions.'s essential to listen to your body and only make dietary changes that make you feel good. Your body's feedback is valuable. If find the content helpful, please consider liking, subscribing, and sharing to help spread the message.

SECTION 2

PRACTICAL GUIDANCE

Ultimate Animal-Products Meal Plan

Introducing the Ultimate Animal Products Meal Plan! Embark on a delectable journey filled with nourishing animal-based foods, perfect for those following a carnivorous dietary lifestyle.

Indulge in an array of tantalizing options such as succulent beef, tender pork, flavorful lamb, and rich, velvety eggs. Elevate your meals with the creamy goodness of butter, an assortment of cheeses, and the savory enhancement of salt.

The Carnivore Experience

Start your day with invigorating breakfasts featuring sizzling bacon, hearty omelets, or delicate smoked salmon. For fulfilling lunches, relish grilled chicken, sumptuous turkey, or seared sea-bass, paired with your favorite cheese.

As the day winds down, treat yourself to mouthwatering dinners starring juicy steak, buttery lobster, or perfectly seared scallops.

Need a quick bite? Snack on cheese bites, hard-boiled eggs, or crispy turkey bacon for a satisfying pick-me-up throughout the day.

Discover the simplicity and indulgence of an exclusively animal products meal plan, designed to tantalize your taste buds while meeting your nutritional needs.

Ditch the complexity and embrace the deliciousness of animal-based feasts!

Day 1

Breakfast

Cheese and Bacon Omelette

Lunch

5 Minute Steak with Optional Egg Yolk

Snack

Cottage Cheese or Pork Rinds or Boiled Eggs

Dinner

Ground Beef Patties

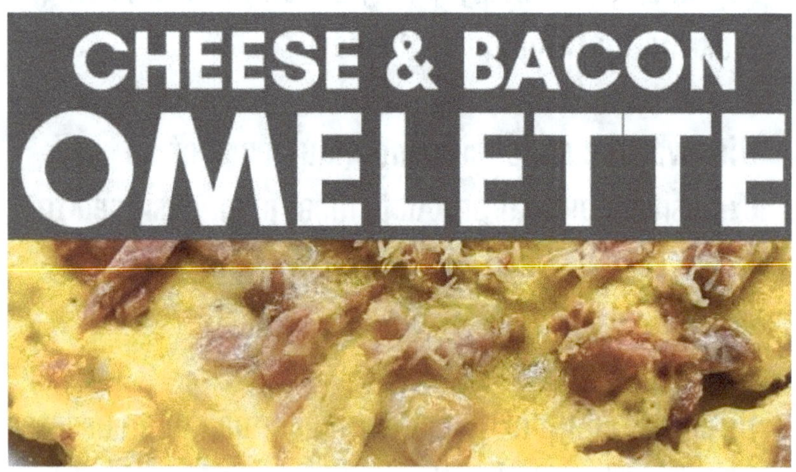

Here's a simple recipe for a cheese and bacon omelette using an air fryer:
Ingredients: -
4 eggs -
Salt to taste -
3 strips of bacon -
Butter -
Shredded cheese of your choice

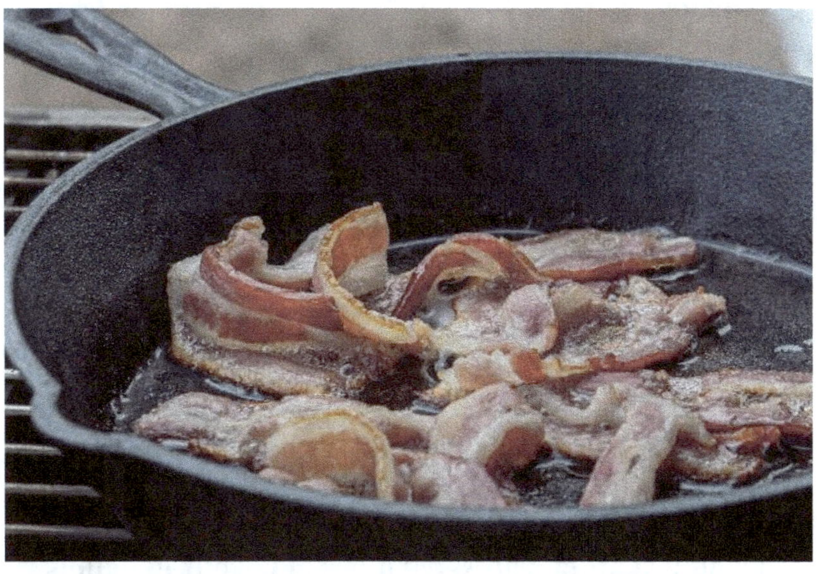

On the next page are the full instructions. If I can cook these meals then ANYONE can!

Instructions:

1. Preheat your air fryer to 350°F (175°C).
2. While the air fryer is preheating, cook the bacon in a skillet until it's crispy. Once cooked, chop the bacon into small pieces and set it aside.
3. In a bowl, beat the eggs and season with salt.
4. Add the chopped bacon to the beaten eggs and mix well.
5. Grease the air fryer basket with butter to prevent sticking.
6. Pour the egg and bacon mixture into the prepared air fryer basket.
7. Cook in the air fryer at 350°F (175°C) for about 8-10 minutes, or until the omelette is set and cooked through.
8. Sprinkle shredded cheese over the omelette and cook for an additional 1-2 minutes, or until the cheese is melted.
9. Carefully remove the omelette from the air fryer using a spatula, and serve hot. Enjoy your delicious cheese and bacon omelette made in the air fryer!

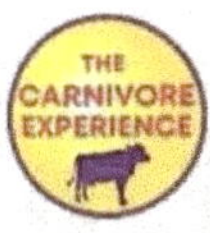

Weekly Meal Planner

Monday

Breakfast	Cheese and Ham Omelette
Lunch	Salmon or pan-fried pork
Dinner	Ground beef patties

Tuesday

Breakfast	Steak and eggs
Lunch	Ribeye steak
Dinner	Chicken thighs

Wednesday

Breakfast	Kefir and two-four eggs
Lunch	Tuna (fresh or canned)
Dinner	Chicken thighs with bacon

Thursday

Breakfast	Poached eggs with bacon
Lunch	Sardines (tinned or fresh)
Dinner	Bone broth & roast chicken

Videos and recipes are available at
www.theukcarnivore.com/meal-plans
Or even better on the Carnivore Experience App

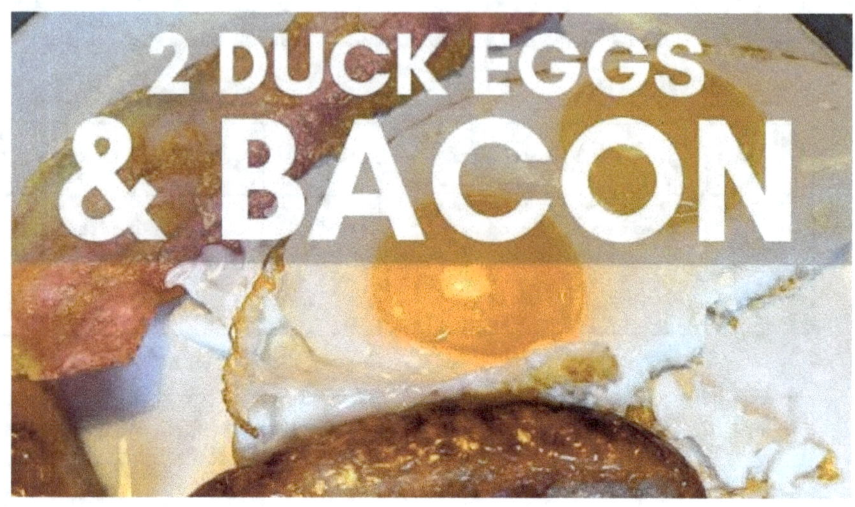

Day 2

Breakfast

Duck Eggs (or Chicken) Bacon and Sausage

Lunch

Surf 'n' Turf Sardines and Beef Burgers

Snack

Butter Bites or Pre-cooked Bacon or Cheese

Dinner

Free Range Roasted Chicken

Remember all of these recipes have videos available on my Carnivore Experience App.

Cooking a breakfast of two duck eggs, sausage, and bacon using a pan and butter only can result in a delicious and hearty morning meal.

Ingredients:
2 duck eggs -
Sausage links or patties -
Bacon strips -
Butter -
Salt and pepper (optional)

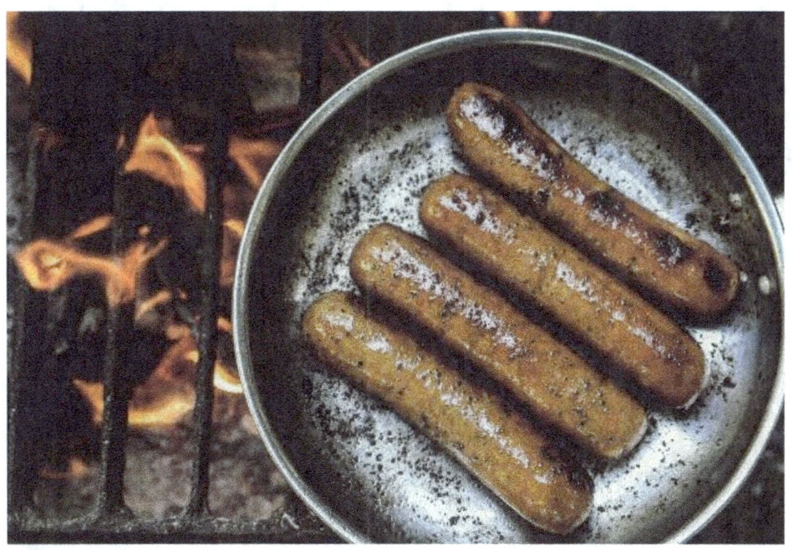

Instructions:

The Carnivore Experience

1. Cook the Bacon and Sausage: Place a large skillet or frying pan over medium heat. Add a small amount of butter to the pan, then add the bacon strips and sausage links or patties. Cook them until they reach the desired level of crispiness and donees, turning occasionally to ensure even cooking.
2. Remove the Bacon and Sausage: Once the bacon and sausage are cooked, use tongs to remove them from the pan and place them on a plate lined with paper towels to drain any excess fat.
3. Cook the Duck Eggs: In the same pan, add a bit more butter if needed, and carefully crack the duck eggs into the pan. Cook them to your desired doneness, whether sunny-side up, over-easy, or any other preferred style.
4. Season the Eggs: If desired, season the eggs with salt and pepper to enhance their flavor, and then remove the pan from the heat.
5. Serve: Plate the cooked duck eggs, sausage, and bacon, and serve them hot for a delicious and satisfying breakfast.

Day 3

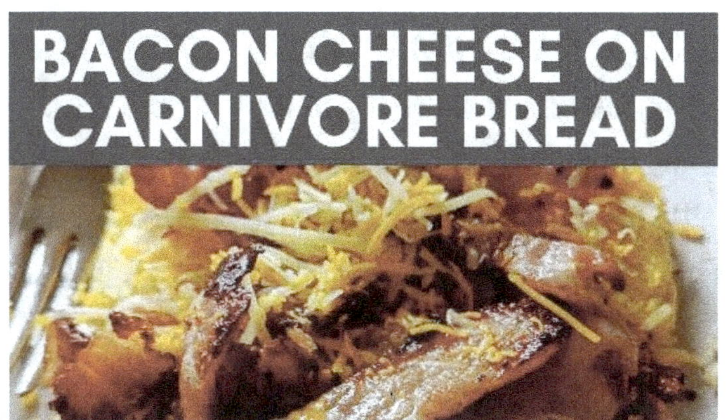

Breakfast

Bacon, Cheese and Carnivore Bread

Lunch

Chicken Thighs with Bacon

Snack

Tuna (fresh or canned)

Dinner

28-Day-Aged Steak

Videos and recipes are available at
www.theukcarnivore.com/meal-plans

Delicious Carnivore Bread Pizza

Learn how to make a mouthwatering carnivore bread / pizza in the online video if you have access to it. There Coach Stephen shows you step by step how to make the carnivore bread using high protein meat powder from Protermars-snacks

2 eggs
1/4 teaspoon of baking powder
and 40 grams of melted butter.

Once the bread is ready, coach Stephen demonstrates how to assemble the 'scruffy' pizza by adding a variety of cheeses and bacon.

The end result is a delectable, cheesy mess that is sure to satisfy your carnivorous cravings! www.protermars-snacks.co.uk is where I obtained the powder

Day 4

Breakfast

Poached Eggs with Bacon and / or Sausage

Lunch

Tuna and Hard Boiled Eggs

Snack

Bone Broth with Chicken Dippers

Dinner

Roasted Leg of Lamb

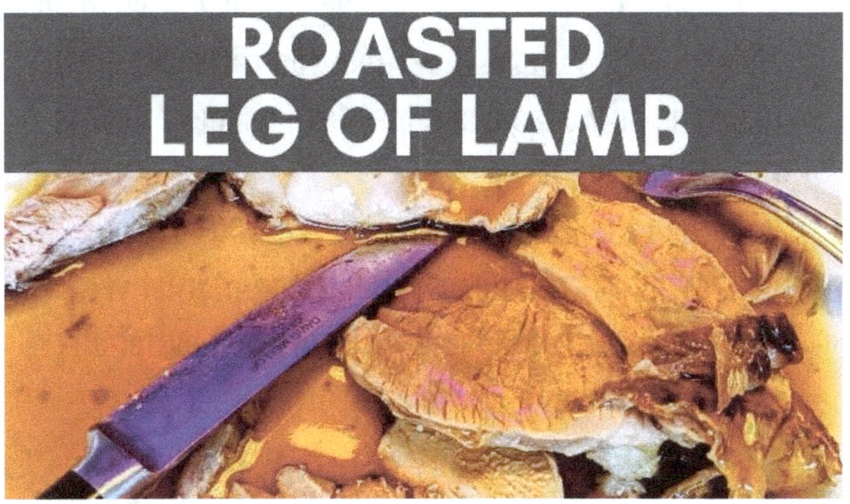

Roasting a leg of lamb with only butter and a sprig of rosemary can result in a delicious and flavorful dish.

Here's a simple guide to prepare the leg of lamb using these minimal ingredients:

Ingredients:

Leg of lamb - Butter - Sprig of rosemary - Salt and pepper (optional)

Instructions:

1. Preheat the Oven: Preheat your oven to 325°F (165°C).

2. Prepare the Leg of Lamb: Place the leg of lamb on a clean work surface. If desired, you can make small incisions in the lamb and insert thin slices of garlic to enhance the flavor.

3. Season the Lamb: Generously season the leg of lamb with salt and pepper if desired. Alternatively, you can also rub the lamb with softened butter all over the surface to create a flavorful crust during roasting.

4. Add Rosemary: Place a sprig of rosemary on top of the leg of lamb.

The aromatic herb will infuse the lamb with a delightful flavor during the roasting process.

5. Place in Roasting Pan: Transfer the seasoned leg of lamb to a roasting pan, and add a few additional small dabs of butter on top of the meat for extra flavor and moisture.

6. Roast the Lamb: Place the roasting pan with the leg of lamb into the preheated oven. Roast the lamb for approximately 20 minutes per pound (about 45 minutes per kilogram) for medium doneness, adjusting the time according to your preferred level of doneness.

7. Baste the Lamb: During the roasting process, baste the leg of lamb with the pan juices and butter every 20-30 minutes to keep it moist and flavorful.

8. Rest and Serve: Once the leg of lamb reaches your desired level of doneness (recommended internal temperature of 145°F or 63°C for medium-rare), remove it from the oven and let it rest for 15-20 minutes before carving.

Resting the meat allows the juices to redistribute, resulting in a tender and flavorful roast.

Day 5

Breakfast

Chicken Livers and Scrambled Eggs

Lunch

Mixed Grill Snack Hard Boiled Eggs

Dinner

T-Bone Steak

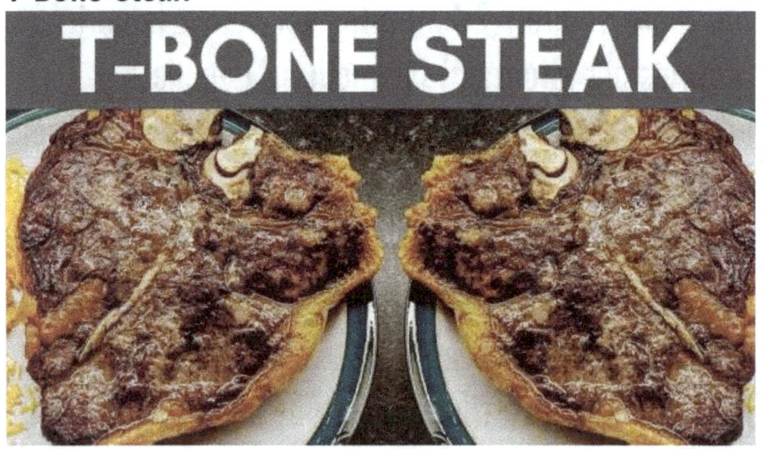

Pan-frying a T-bone steak with only butter and salt can create a delicious and flavorful dish.

On the next page there's a simple guide to pan-fry a T-Bone steak using minimal ingredients

The Carnivore Experience

Ingredients:
- T-bone steak
- Butter
- Salt

Instructions:

1. Preparing the Steak: Remove the T-bone steak from the refrigerator and let it sit at room temperature for about 30 minutes to ensure even cooking. Pat the steak dry with paper towels to remove any excess moisture. Season both sides of the steak with salt, ensuring even coverage.

2. Preheat the Pan: Place a heavy-bottomed skillet or frying pan over medium-high heat and allow it to preheat. Make sure the pan is hot before adding the steak.

3. Add Butter: Once the pan is hot, add a generous amount of butter to the pan. You want enough butter to coat the bottom of the pan and create a sizzling, flavorful base for the steak.

4. Searing the Steak: Carefully place the seasoned T-bone steak in the hot pan.

Let the steak sear undisturbed for about 3-4 minutes on each side, or until a golden-brown crust forms.

5. Basting with Butter: As the steak cooks, use a spoon to continually baste the steak with the melted butter from the pan. This will infuse the steak with rich flavor and help keep it moist.

6. Checking for Doneness: Use a meat thermometer to check For a medium-rare T-bone steak, aim for an internal temperature of 130-135°F (54-57°C), and for a medium steak, aim for 140-145°F (60-63°C).

7. Rest and Serve: Once the steak reaches your preferred level of doneness, remove it from the pan and let it rest for a few minutes before slicing. This resting period allows the juices to redistribute, resulting in a tender and flavorful steak.

Day 6

Breakfast

Chicken and Feta Omelette

Lunch

Lamb Roast (around 2pm...possibly start a fast)

Snack

If you can leave them today, then do!

Dinner

Try to skip dinner unless you are very hungry

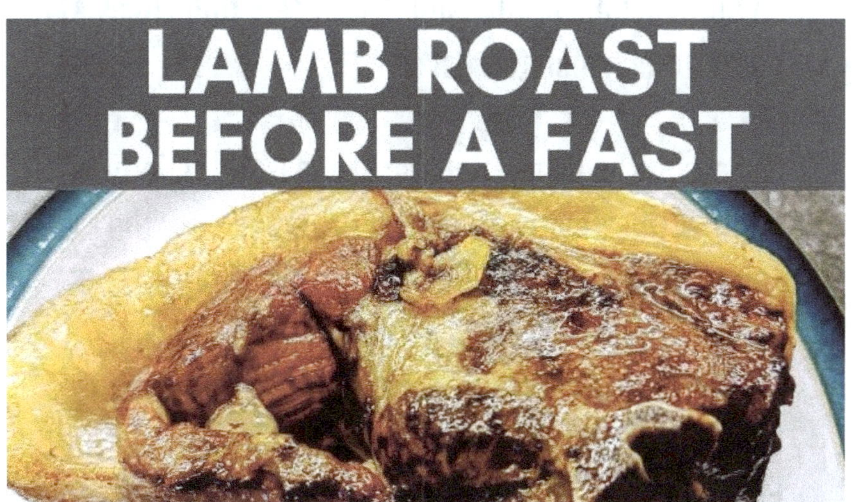

Here's a simple guide to roasting a joint of lamb using these minimal ingredients:

Ingredients:

Joint of lamb - Butter - Salt - Optional: Garlic (for added flavor)

Instructions:

1. Preheat the Oven: Preheat your oven to 325°F (160°C).

2. Prepare the Lamb: Take the joint of lamb and pat it dry with paper towels. If desired, you can make small incisions in the lamb and insert thin slices of garlic to enhance the flavor.

3. Season the Lamb: Generously season the joint of lamb with salt, ensuring even coverage over the surface of the meat.

4. Add Butter: Place the joint of lamb in a roasting pan. Using your hands or a spoon, spread softened butter all over the surface of the lamb. The butter will help create a flavorful crust and keep the meat moist during the roasting process.

5. Roast the Lamb: Place the roasting pan with the lamb into the preheated oven. Roast the lamb for approximately 20 minutes per pound (about 45 minutes per kilogram) for medium doneness, adjusting the time according to your preferred level of doneness.

6. Baste the Lamb: During the roasting process, baste the lamb with the melted butter and pan juices every 20-30 minutes to keep it moist and flavorful.

7. Check for Doneness: Use a meat thermometer to check for the desired level of doneness. For a medium-rare joint of lamb, aim for an internal temperature of 145°F (63°C), and for a medium joint of lamb, aim for 160°F (71°C).

8. Rest and Serve: Once the joint of lamb reaches your preferred level of doneness, remove it from the oven and let it rest for at least 15-20 minutes before carving.

Day 7

Breakfast
(Wait as long as you can before eating) Scrambled
Eggs with Mozzarella
Lunch-Skipped
Snack
Steak Bites
Dinner
Sea-Bass and Steak

To combine sea bass cooked in a pan with butter and
a steak cooked in an air fryer with salt, you can
create a surf and turf meal. See the next page.

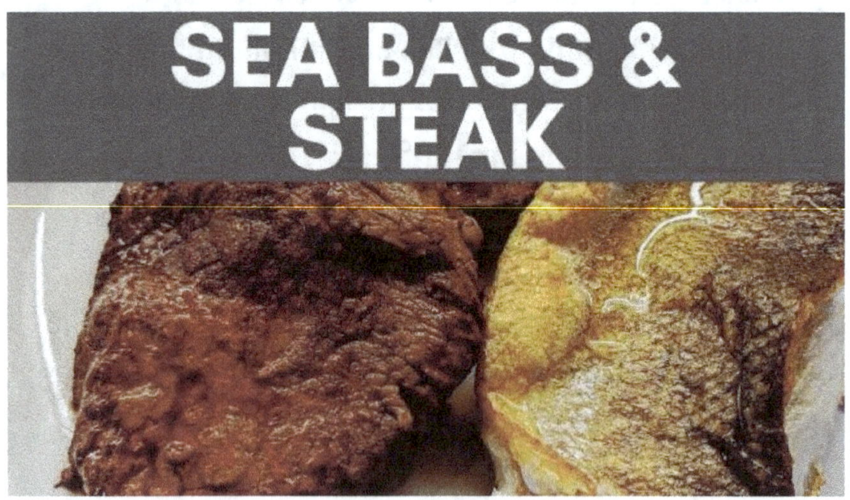

Here's how you can prepare both the sea bass and the steak in the respective cooking methods, and then combine them for a delicious meal: Cooking Sea Bass with Butter in a Pan:

Ingredients:
Sea bass fillets - Butter - Salt - Lemon (optional)
Instructions:
1. Pat the sea bass fillets dry with paper towels and season them with salt on both sides.

2. In a preheated pan, melt a generous amount of butter over medium-high heat.

3. Once the butter is melted and sizzling, carefully place the sea bass fillets in the pan, skin side down.

4. Cook the sea bass for about 4-5 minutes on each side, or until the fillets are cooked through and the skin is crisp and golden.

5. Optional: Squeeze some fresh lemon juice over the cooked sea bass for added flavor.

Cooking the Steak with Salt in an Air Fryer:

Ingredients: - Steak - Salt
Instructions:

1. Preheat the air fryer to 400°F (200°C) for a few minutes.
2. Season the steak generously with salt on both sides.
3. Place the seasoned steak in the air fryer basket and cook it for about 10-14 minutes, depending on the desired level of doneness.

Combining the Sea Bass and Steak:

Once both the sea bass and steak are cooked, you can arrange them on a serving platter for a beautiful surf and turf presentation.

Serve the sea bass fillets alongside the air-fried steak, allowing guests to enjoy both delicious proteins in one amazing meal.

Day 8

Breakfast

Scrambled or Poached Eggs and Bacon

Lunch

Salmon or Pan-Fried Pork

Snack

Cottage Cheese or Pork Rinds or Boiled Eggs

Dinner

Beef Rib Joint or Surf 'n' Turf (Sardines and Beef)

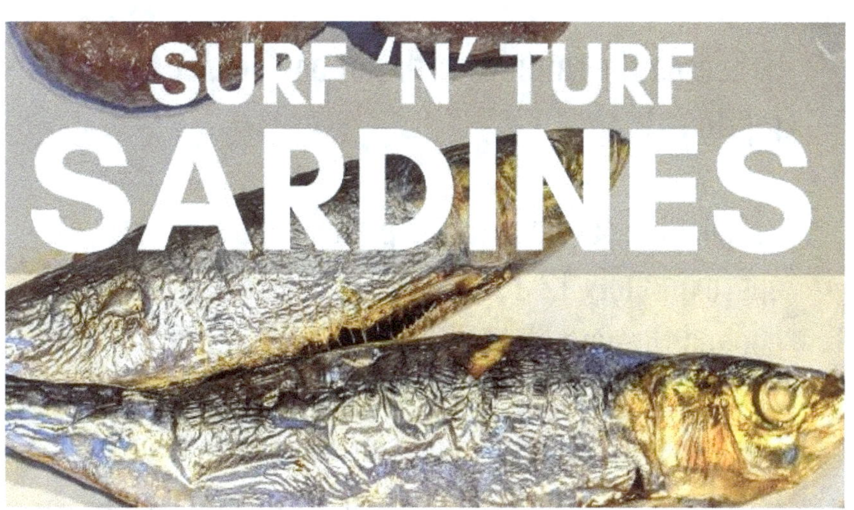

Ingredients: - Fresh sardines
Instructions:
1. Preheat your oven to 400°F (200°C).

2. Rinse the fresh sardines under cold water and pat them dry with paper towels.

3. Place the sardines on a baking sheet lined with parchment paper or lightly greased.

4. You could add a blob of butter to the sardines if you wish, ensuring they are coated evenly.

5. Season the sardines with salt and pepper to taste (optional)

6. Bake the sardines in the preheated oven for approximately 12-15 minutes, or until they are cooked through and easily flake with a fork.

Once they are cooked, you can serve with your beef burgers or you could have them as they are! Enjoy your delicious and nutritious meal!

To cook fresh beef burgers in an oven fryer:

1. Preheat the Oven Air Fryer: Preheat your oven air fryer to the recommended temperature, typically around 375-400°F (190-200°C).

2. Prepare the Beef Burgers: Form the fresh beef into burger patties, season them with salt (or pepper.)

3. Preheat the Oven Air Fryer Basket: Preheat the basket for 2 minutes to ensure even cooking.

4. Place the Burgers in the Air Fryer Basket: Place the patties in the air fryer basket, leaving space between each patty.

5. Cook the Burgers: Cook the burgers for about 9-12 minutes, depends on the thickness. It's a good idea to flip them halfway through to ensure even browning.

6. Check for Doneness: Use a meat thermometer to check the internal temperature of the burgers.

The USDA recommends cooking ground beef to an internal temperature of 160°F (71°C) for safety.

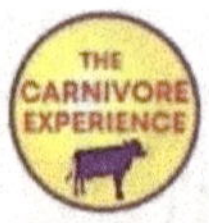

Weekly Meal Planner

Monday

Breakfast	Cheese and Ham Omelette
Lunch	Salmon or pan-fried pork
Dinner	Ground beef patties

Tuesday

Breakfast	Steak and eggs
Lunch	Ribeye steak
Dinner	Chicken thighs

Wednesday

Breakfast	Kefir and two-four eggs
Lunch	Tuna (fresh or canned)
Dinner	Chicken thighs with bacon

Thursday

Breakfast	Poached eggs with bacon
Lunch	Sardines (tinned or fresh)
Dinner	Bone broth & roast chicken

Friday

Breakfast	Chicken livers & scrambled eggs
Lunch	Pork chops
Dinner	Turkey burgers

Saturday

Breakfast	Chicken and feta omelette
Lunch	Slow roasted salmon
Dinner	Beef liver or Ground beef, butter and eggs

Sunday

Breakfast	Eggs (scrambled or poached) and bacon
Lunch	Cottage cheese or pork rinds or boiled eggs
Dinner	Ground beef patties

Notes

"This serves as an illustrative meal plan, and personalized ones are provided upon booking a coaching session."

Exploring the Carnivore Experience App

Unlocking Content, Tracking Progress &
Engaging with Members
Discover the features and benefits of
the Carnivore Experience app

There are various sections of the app, including FREE access the Secrets Course, or an upgrade to the Carnivore Science course.

Join in the 30 Day Kickstart program or the 30 Plus Advantage for those who want additional support on their carnivore journey.

Explore the community tab to connect with like-minded individuals and participate in discussions on food, health concerns, and more.

Plus, use the tracking feature which allows you to monitor your progress and customize your experience on the app.

Immerse yourself in the carnivore lifestyle with this comprehensive app!

DOWNLOAD THE CARNIVORE EXPERIENCE APP

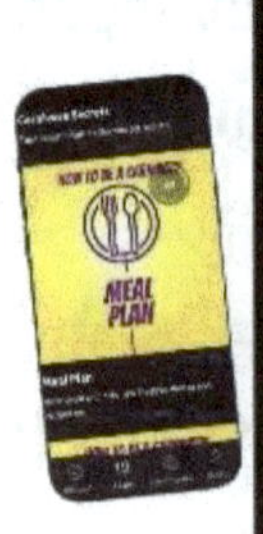

Meal Frequency

How often should you eat?

OMAD and 2MAD (what do they mean?)
What are the pro's and cons of eating one meal a day?

Eating one meal a day, also known as the "one meal a day" **(OMAD)**, is a type of intermittent fasting where a person only eats during a specific time window and fasts for the remaining hours of the day.

OMAD
one meal a day

Eating one meal a day, also known as OMAD, is a type of intermittent fasting where a person only eats during a specific time window and fasts for the remaining hours of the day.

Pros of eating one meal a day
Increased insulin sensitivity: Intermittent fasting has been shown to increase insulin sensitivity, which can be beneficial for people with type 2 diabetes.

Improved digestion: By eating one large meal per day, it may lead to better digestion compared to eating multiple smaller meals throughout the day.

Increased focus and mental clarity: Intermittent fasting has been associated with improved brain function and increased focus.

Better blood glucose control: You are not inputting nutrients into your system over the entire day blood glucose management should be easier.

Less food preparation & clean up time: Only cook once a day, only clean up once a day

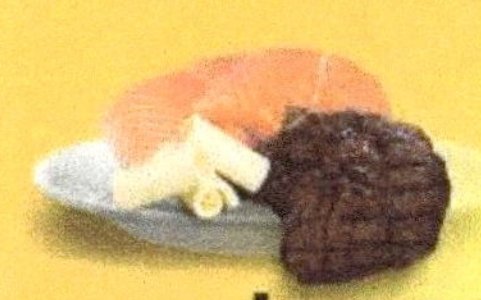

**OMAD
PROS**

- Increased insulin sensitivity
- Improved digestion
- Increased focus and mental clarity
- Better blood glucose control
- Less food preparation and clean up

Cons of eating one meal a day:
Difficult to eat enough:: By only eating one meal a day, it can be difficult to get all of the necessary nutrients the body needs, especially proteins and fats.

Hunger and cravings: Eating only one meal a day can lead to intense hunger and cravings, which can be difficult to resist.

Decreased energy levels: Eating one large meal can cause a spike in blood sugar followed by a rapid decrease, leading to decreased energy levels and fatigue.

Increased risk of binge eating: Restricting food intake to only one meal per day may lead to overeating or binge eating during that meal.

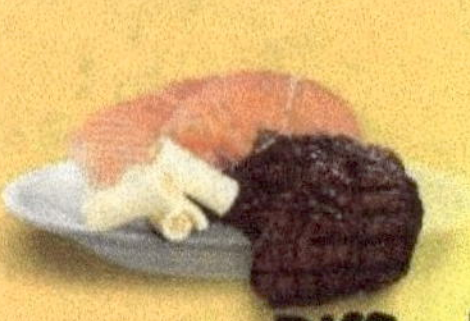

Unsustainable: Eating One Meal A Day may be difficult for some to maintain in the long term and could lead to feelings of deprivation in others. Many people do report loving it though!

Anti-social in some families: If eating is a social event with the children or partner etc.

ONE MEAL A DAY

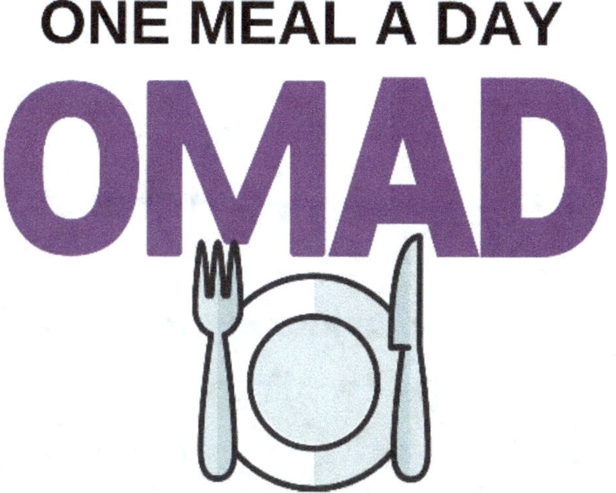

It's important to note that the "one meal a day" diet is not suitable for everyone and may not be recommended for individuals with certain health conditions, such as diabetes, or for athletes and active individuals who have high energy and protein requirements.

Two Meals A Day (2MAD)

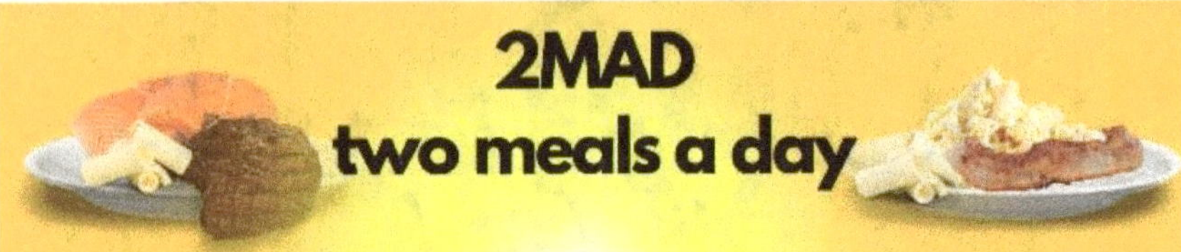

Pros of eating two meals a day:

Improved digestion: By eating two larger meals per day instead of multiple smaller meals, it may lead to better digestion compared to eating multiple smaller meals throughout the day.

The Carnivore Experience

Increased focus and mental clarity: Intermittent fasting has been associated with improved brain function and increased focus.

Flexibility: The two meals a day diet allows for more flexibility compared to the "one meal a day" diet, which can be more difficult to maintain in the long term.

Easier to eat enough: Especially protein and fats
More Socially Accepted: May fit in better with family life.

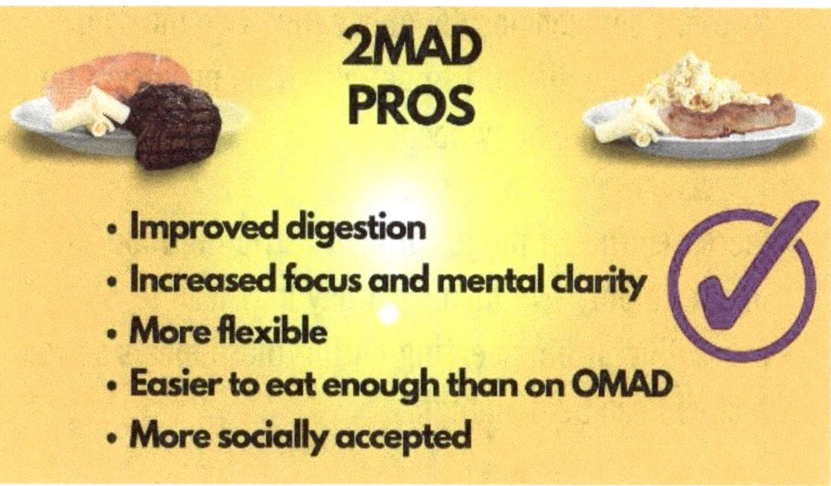

Cons of eating two meals a day:
Hunger and cravings: For some you still might not be able to eat enough food, can lead to intense hunger and cravings, which can be difficult to resist. You may also be unable to digest the fat in the quantity you need while healing

Decreased energy levels: Eating two large meals can, in some people, cause spikes in blood sugar followed by rapid decreases, leading to decreased energy levels and fatigue.

Nutrient deficiencies: By only eating two meals a day, it can be difficult to get all of the necessary fat and protein the body needs.

Increased risk of binge eating: Restricting food intake to only two meals per day may lead to overeating or binge eating during those meals as you feel you can't eat enough.

Unsustainable: This diet may be difficult for some people to maintain in the long term and could lead to feelings of deprivation.

It's important to note that the "two meals a day" diet is not suitable for everyone and may not be recommended for individuals with certain health conditions, such as diabetes, or for athletes and active individuals who have high energy requirements.

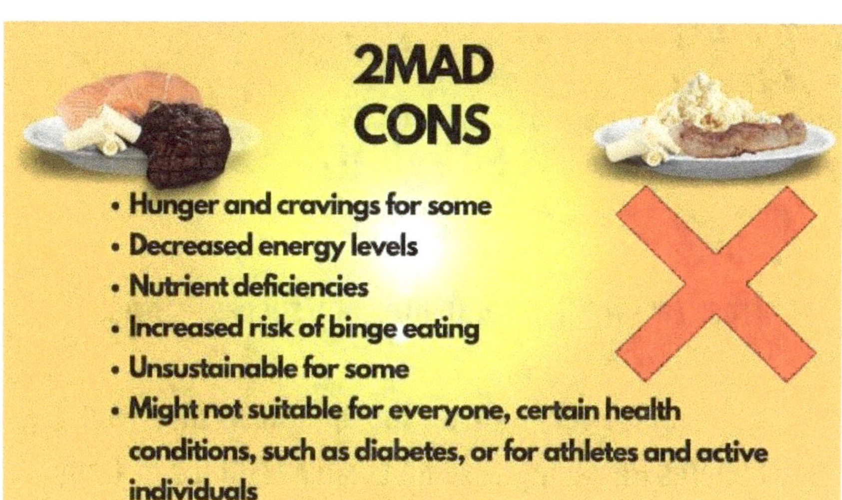

The Carnivore Experience

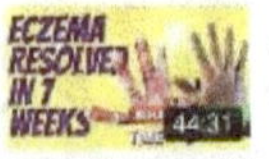

A Lifetime of Eczema Resolved in 7 Weeks...
Growing up, Bradley had some terrible skin issues. Eczema plagued him his whole life, almost since birth. But it wasn't un...

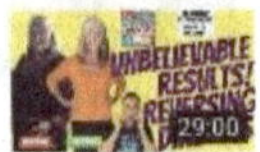

Unbelievable Results! Reversing Diabetes and Losing Body...
Are you ready to be inspired by an incredible health journey? In this video, we're sharing the amazing story of Connie, who...

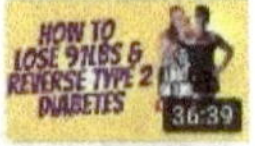

From Severe Joint Pain to London Marathon: A Neuroscien...
In this episode, we had the pleasure of speaking with Sara, a neuroscientist working for the NHS, about her truly remarkabl...

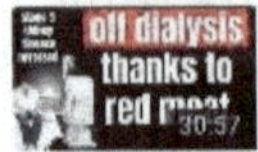

Incredible Recovery: From Stage 5 Kidney Disease to Healt...
Join us as we delve into the extraordinary story of Eric, who defied all odds by reversing his stage 5 kidney disease natural...

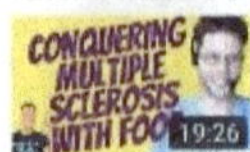

Overcoming Chronic Disease: How One Man Transformed ...
Are you ready for an inspiring and uplifting story? Meet Kevin, a man who was once told he would live with chronic progressiv...

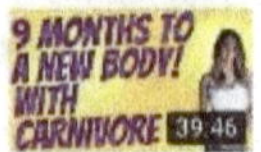

Dr. Solt: Unleashing the Power of Carnivore: A Transformat...
Prepare to be captivated as we dive deep into an incredible interview with the esteemed Dr. Sabrina Solt. In this eye-...

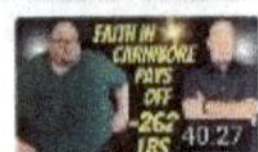

262lb Fat Loss, Reversed Fatty Liver, Lower Blood Pressur...
Shawn White updated fat loss 23/7/2023 is now 262lbs! Detailed Summary: 262lb Fat Loss, Reversed Fatty Liver, Lowe...

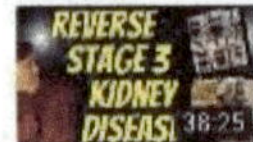

Rebirth Through Ribeyes: Amy's Remarkable Recovery with...
In my recent interview with 'Carnivore Diet Amy', her transformative journey with the carnivore diet was unveiled....

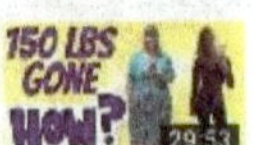

150lb Fat Loss Success Story will HELP you lose weight!
In this video, I'm sharing the story of Emily's 150lb fat loss with you. We'll tell you how Emily lost weight and kept it off using a...

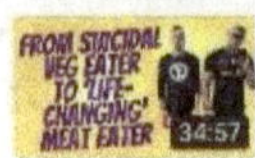

Carnivore Diet Transformed My Life: From Depression and ...
In this compelling interview, we meet Trevor Griffith, a man who has transformed his life through the carnivore diet. For years,...

SUCCESS STORIES Over 150 Video success stories Over 1,000 written reviews

https://www.theukcarnivore.com/success-stories

You can also see more on the app. Reversing Type 2 Diabetes Resolving Eczema Losing >100 lbs of Body Fat Getting of Medication Healing Kidneys Dealing With Depression And so much more. All true stories.

DANKE!
THANK YOU!
MERCI!
GRAZIE!
GRACIAS!
DANK JE WEL!

. . . .

Thank you to everyone who has purchased my book
"How to Be Carnivore:
Your Roadmap to Better Health."

Your support and interest mean a great deal to me, and I am sincerely grateful for your readership. I am excited to announce that I am currently working on another book which will provide insights into the interpretation of blood tests within the context of a carnivore diet. I look forward to sharing this valuable information with you, and I appreciate your continued support on this journey to better health.

Coach Stephen BSc. (Hons.)

Guide To Blood Tests

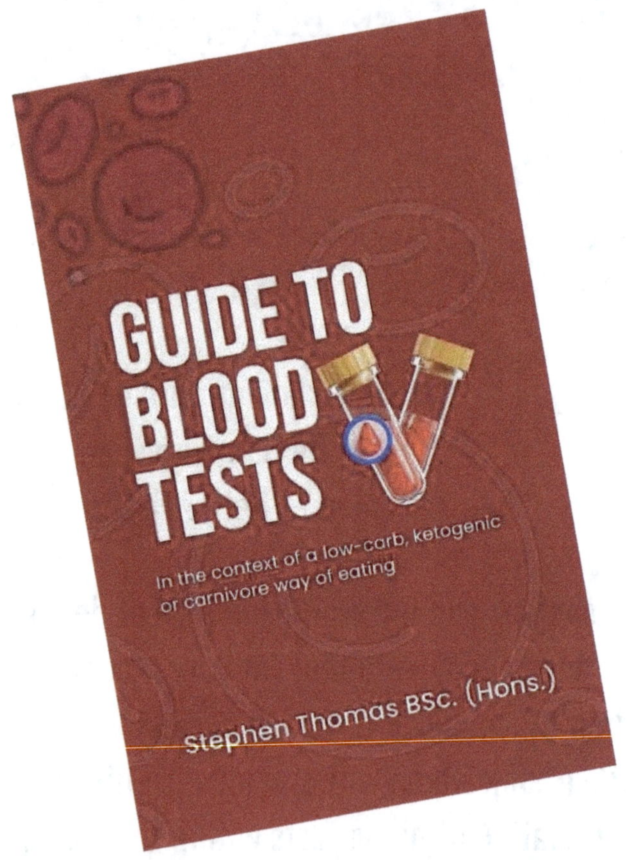

Buy it now
https://stan.store/Carnivoredietresults/p/bloods-book

Carb-Free Muscle Growth

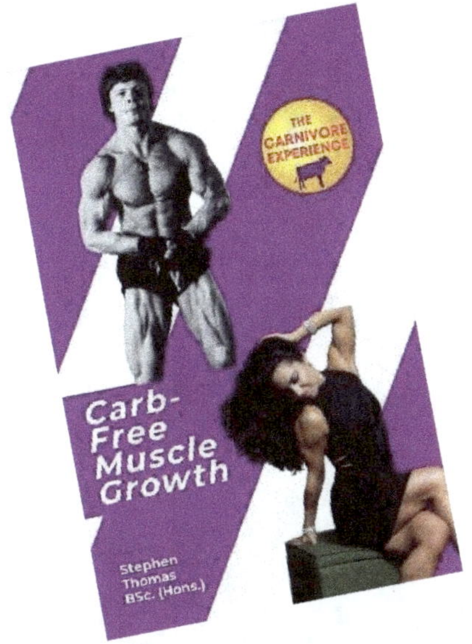

The purpose of my book is to dispel the myth that muscle building is reliant on carbohydrates. Despite the prevailing belief, thousands of individuals have successfully built muscle without carbohydrates, some even achieving victory in bodybuilding competitions.

It's essential to recognize that muscle is primarily composed of protein, and fat serves as an ample source of energy. Contrary to popular belief, there is no such thing as an essential carbohydrate.